Confronting Traumatic Brain Injury

William J. Winslade

Confronting

Traumatic

Brain Injury

DEVASTATION,

HOPE, AND

HEALING

Yale University Press
New Haven & London

Designed by Nancy Ovedovitz and set in Adobe Garamond type by Tseng Information Systems, Inc. Printed in the United States of America by Vail-Ballou Press, Binghamton, New York.

Library of Congress Cataloging-in-Publication Data

Winslade, William J.
Confronting traumatic brain injury : devastation, hope, and healing / William J. Winslade.
    p.   cm.
Includes bibliographical references and index.
ISBN 0-300-07026-8
1. Brain damage—Popular works.
2. Head—Wounds and injuries—Popular works.   I. Title.
RC387.5.W55   1998
617.4′81044—dc21   97-32406

A catalogue record for this book is available from the British Library.

The paper in this book meets the guidelines for permanence and durability of the Committee on Production Guidelines for Book Longevity of the Council on Library Resources.

10 9 8 7 6 5 4 3 2

For my mother, Lillian B. Key, and my late grandmother,
Anna B. Schneider

Contents

Foreword

Few things are more powerful than the written word. A book can best be described as a vessel carrying the author's thoughts, dreams, hopes, and ideas, communicated in written form. The beauty of a book is that these thoughts, dreams, hopes, and ideas then move into the public domain, becoming available for the edification of anyone who desires further knowledge. Few things are more enduring than the written word. Triumphing over mortality, an author's work remains as a testament to life.

With that in mind, I would like to put pen to paper and compose a foreword for a book that I consider a must-read. Using a masterful blend of first-person accounts, statistics, and research, *Confronting Traumatic Brain Injury: Devastation, Hope, and Healing* recognizes the immeasurable consequences that brain injury has on both a human and an economic scale. Not only does William J. Winslade attest to the realities faced by all individuals and their families who have been affected by brain injuries, but he also outlines a multifaceted plan of action to increase our awareness of what brain injury is and how we can prevent it.

In a persuasive and forthright manner, Winslade details the unfortunate lack of a general public awareness about brain injury, while explaining that this health crisis kills or disables more children and young adults than does any other single cause. To counteract the widespread knowledge gap and pervasive ambivalence surrounding the subject of brain injury, Winslade encourages a shift in attitude. In Chapter 10, he mentions how Lyndon Johnson once noted that each year more Americans were killed on the highway than died in the entire eleven years of the Vietnam War. Yet American citizens who were critical of U.S. involvement in Vietnam were so vocal in their protests and petitions that they changed not only public policy but cultural opinion as well. Figuratively, this is what brain injury requires—a new march on Washington to quell the epidemic that is claiming or altering the lives of far too many.

Winslade is an avid proponent of sound public policy for reducing the impact of the epidemic, and this agenda is a key factor in differentiating *Confronting Traumatic Brain Injury* from its predecessors. Winslade offers many concrete solutions, not only in the area of assisting those with brain injuries but also in the area of prevention: increasing investment in basic and clinical research, redirecting research efforts to look beyond medical treatment and to focus on rehabilitation, proper training of service providers, meshing broad federal guidelines with state latitude in instituting programs for providing and regulating brain injury–related services, establishing graduated licensing programs for young drivers, preventing concussions among athletes, and legislating gun control that protects our citizens, to name a few.

As vice chairman of the Brain Injury Association, I am heartened to see many of the issues that our organization actively promotes championed here so eloquently. *Confronting Traumatic Brain Injury* moves beyond preaching to the choir to speak to a diverse cross-section of individuals. Brain injury should be a topic of concern for all Americans, and this book makes great strides in achieving that goal.

James S. Brady
Washington, D.C.

Preface

Traumatic brain injury ranks among the most serious public health problems facing the United States and the rest of the developed world. In terms of money, emotional anguish, practical limitations, and lost opportunities, the costs to the brain-injured and their families are enormous and often overwhelming. And because few individuals, even with insurance, can afford high-technology acute treatment and lengthy rehabilitation, we all share the financial burden.

As individuals, each of us is vulnerable to traumatic brain injury. Yet as a society, we are barely beginning to recognize and discuss what is virtually an epidemic of brain injury. Public, private, and institutional responses have been at best sporadic and uneven, and at worst, irresponsible.

Public awareness is the first step to reducing the damage that traumatic brain injury does to individuals and to all of us collectively. I aim here to promote that awareness and to recommend specific measures that we can take to combat and deal with the epidemic. This book describes in plain language what traumatic brain injury is, how it is caused, and what can be done to respond to and prevent it. The closing chapters set out what steps I feel we must take immediately and what long-range goals I think we can hope to achieve. Although we will never eliminate brain injury, we can do much to reduce both its occurrence and its devastation.

In recent years, a number of helpful volumes have been published for professionals who treat and families who live with victims of brain injuries. I hope this book will contribute something useful to these people by putting the epidemic in a larger social, legal, economic, and ethical context.

But I am writing also for a broader audience. Any of us who drives a car or truck, rides a bicycle or motorcycle, plays sports, rears children, has elderly parents, or pays taxes has a vital self-interest in reducing the unacceptably high incidence of traumatic brain injury. We also share a stake in assuring that those who do become its victims receive the treatment that they need in order to reach their maximum potential for self-sufficiency. Anyone involved in education, health care, legislation, municipal government, or law enforcement has an even greater need to become informed on this crucial topic. Defeating the epidemic of brain injury requires specific public policy initiatives combined with systematic changes in cultural attitudes and personal behavior. This book proposes and explains them.

Some of my suggestions may prompt controversy. So much the better. The broader the discussion of traumatic brain injury, the greater the potential benefits for us all.

Acknowledgments

Russell Moody, whose brain injury is described later, was the inspiration for this book, and he brought me back in touch with my own childhood experiences as a victim of traumatic brain injury. The cooperation and generous financial support of the Moody Foundation gave me the time to research the subject. Both Russell Moody and his father, Robert "Bobby" Moody, Jr., shared their insights into the challenges faced by the brain-injured and their families. They also made Russell's medical and rehabilitation records available to me. Their candor and their personal courage and determination helped to give this book human depth. Peter Moore and Bernice Torregrossa of the Moody Foundation, along with the staff of the Transitional Learning Center, provided essential encouragement and information.

After my own very early traumatic brain injury (which I recount in the Introduction), Dr. Max Bernauer, the staff at the hospital where I was treated, and the private-duty nurses who watched over me during my recovery enabled my brain to heal. My family took care of me, paid my hospital bills, and provided the supportive environment that a small child needs, along with good medical care, in order to recover from severe head trauma. Victor Werp and Adeline Werp provided valuable letters and other documentation about my injury and its aftermath.

Numerous students, researchers, and colleagues have contributed in many ways to this book. David Barnard suggested that I participate in a conference on neurotrauma, a meeting that launched my professional interest in brain injury and prompted me to reconstruct my own case. Richard Weiner arranged the CT scan and Melvyn Schreiber provided the MRI images that showed me the effects of my injury on my skull and brain. Joe Tabaracci collaborated with me on an early article about prognosis in head injury. The Lutheran General Hospital Department of Pediatrics, thanks to Prudy Krieger, gave me an opportunity to present some of my early work on brain injury. Howard Brody and his colleagues from Michigan State University's Medical Humanities Program gave me an opportunity to present some of my preliminary thoughts at a summer seminar on bioethics.

Considerable background material for this book was compiled by Mary Finch, Phil Head, S. Van McCrary, Kayhan Parsi, Pau Rana, and Kristi Schrode as well as other students at the University of Texas Medical Branch at Galveston and the University of Houston Law Center. Catherine Bontke, Howard Eisenberg, Ralph Frankowski, Bryan Jennett, Harvey Levin, and Richard Weiner were among the specialists who helped me to learn about the treatment of traumatic brain injury. Barbara Bowers, Pam Harmann, Katie Matlack, and Al Vaiani informed me about the emergency, acute, and chronic care of head-injured patients.

Ron Carson, my other colleagues, and my students at the Institute for the Medical Humanities continually provided stimulation, insight, criticism, and opportunities for conversation that made my work enjoyable and productive. The staff at the institute—especially Stacey Gottlob, Sharon Goodwin, and the late Betty Herman—supported my efforts by carrying out administrative and secretarial responsibilities with efficiency, patience, and good humor. Mark Rothstein, other colleagues, and students at the University of Houston Health Law and Policy Institute challenged me to understand the legal, ethical, and policy implications of my work. Göran Lantz and other colleagues at the Ersta Institute for Medical Ethics in Stockholm, Sweden, generously shared their ideas with me. The two months that I spent at the Ersta Institute in 1993 gave me not only much-needed time for reflection about this book but also a chance to learn about how Swedish society reduces brain injury through safety measures and effective public transportation.

The National Head Injury Foundation, now known as the Brain Injury Association, supplied me with much information and many contacts both when I began and as I continued my research; George Zitnay and Sue Guzman were especially cooperative. Interviews with Dan Beauchamp, Gerald Bush, Eric Engum, Marilyn Spivak, and William D. Willis helped me to appreciate the enormous extent of the head injury epidemic. Many other brain-injury volunteers and professionals, including John Banja, Walter R. M. High, Don Lehmkuhl, William Reynolds, and David Seaton, educated me about various aspects of brain trauma. Dan Fox assisted me as I thought through important problems, and he suggested several avenues for further research.

I am grateful to the Rockwell Fund in Houston for essential research support. James L. and Charlene Pate and the Pennzoil Foundation provided support for research. The Rockefeller Foundation, the Greenwall Foundation, the Park Ridge Center, the Institute for the Medical Humanities, the University of Texas Medical Branch at Galveston, and the University of Texas Chancellor's Office generously supported my organizing of an international conference on permanently unconscious patients, held at the Bellagio Conference Center in Italy in 1994. The Rockefeller Foundation also supported the work of Roger Haile, a superb and sensitive photographer who documented the recovery of the head injury victim who appears in this book under the pseudonym Donny Michaels. I am immensely grateful to this patient and to his family for sharing their experiences and ideas with me.

Sandy Sheehy's editorial talent and organizational genius enabled me to convert my manuscript and notes into a coherent book. Without her contribution this project could not have been completed. Josh Dubler and Joanna Winslade offered a careful and detailed commentary on the penultimate draft of the manuscript. Their thoughtful suggestions led to numerous improvements in the text. Denise Webb's research on legal, policy, and public health issues provided essential information; she also made numerous valuable editorial suggestions, helped to compile the bibliography, and carefully proofread the entire manuscript. Tom Curtis not only offered excellent editorial assistance in the final stages of the project but also raised key questions that enabled me to clarify my ideas. Sara Clausen and Ethan Carrier gave valuable editorial, research, and bibliographical assistance for the final draft. Marcia Winslade diligently prepared the index.

Warren Carrier, Ron Carson, Deborah Cummins, Sharon Goodwin, Lillian Key, Katie Matlack, S. Van McCrary, Judy Ross, Al Stern, Jack and Dolores Winslade, and Stuart Youngner read some or all of the manuscript and offered valuable suggestions. Joan Lang read and critiqued early as well as later drafts. Chuck and Muriel Lang supplied several pertinent stories about brain injury.

My agent, John Thornton, gave me guidance and good advice at various stages in the completion of the book. At Yale University Press, acquiring editor Jean Thomson Black offered both encouragement and important suggestions for improving the manuscript at every stage. Brenda Kolb's superb editing enhanced the flow of the text and helped me to clarify numerous details. The anonymous reviewers for the press also made helpful comments.

Throughout this project, Joan Lang and my daughters, Joanna and Marcia, gave me their continual support. They listened again and again to my ideas about traumatic brain injury. Their insightful questions, comments, and criticisms were especially valuable when I was trying to think through various puzzles and policy issues. They all contributed suggestions that made this a clearer and more readable book.

Introduction: It Can Happen to Anyone

On September 7, 1943, when I was not quite two, I fell from a second-story back porch and landed headfirst on the concrete pavement. No one saw it happen. My grandmother, who cared for me while my mother was at work, had stepped away momentarily to gather the wash and take it down to the laundry room. When she returned a few moments later, she saw me lying in a pool of blood on the concrete below. Terrified, she hurried down, picked me up, and carried me to Max Bernauer, a gentle Viennese-born family physician who kept his office in our Chicago neighborhood. He had me transported to a nearby hospital.

When my mother arrived at my bedside, she was horrified at the sight. My face was black and blue from the neck up, and my head was so swollen that it looked twice its normal size. Although Dr. Bernauer wanted to be reassuring, he had to admit that he couldn't predict whether I'd live or die. But he took one step that made all the difference in my future: he placed a shunt inside my skull to drain the excess cerebrospinal fluid that a serious head injury generates. That simple plastic tube reduced pressure on my brain and diminished the swelling. Without the shunt, the uncontrolled buildup of fluid—a process called hydrocephalus or, more commonly, water on the brain—would have pressed ever more firmly against the part of the brain stem that regulates breathing. And that could have been fatal.

Dr. Bernauer prescribed little else but patience. He told my parents that nothing could be done apart from watching me closely, one day at a time, to see whether I would survive, whether complications would develop, and whether and how much I'd recover. If I lived, Dr. Bernauer cautioned, I might suffer lifelong mental, emotional, or physical disabilities. For now, I would need to lie perfectly still. Because I'd regained consciousness shortly after the accident, I was given a cherry-flavored red-liquid sedative to keep me quiet and comfortable. I also required my own private-duty nurse round the clock.

Once I had survived the initial trauma, Dr. Bernauer removed bone fragments from the area where my skull had fractured. He decided against installing a metal plate, leaving a portion of my brain protected only by my scalp. High on my head, above and slightly forward of my left ear, I now have an indentation about three inches long and one inch wide—roughly the size of my forefinger.

After five weeks, I left the hospital with no apparent handicaps. Good fortune and low-technology but diligent care had spared me the seizures, headaches, and other disabilities that afflict many victims of head injuries. I didn't need any further rehabilitation. My biggest problem was that, after being bedridden for so long, I had forgotten how to walk and had to relearn that skill.

My mother and father, who'd been having financial difficulties even before my accident, had borrowed the money to pay for my care. My five weeks in the hospital and the doctor's and nurses' bills came to thirteen hundred dollars—a sobering sum in 1943, although it amounts to only about eleven thousand dollars in 1998 dollars. Treatment for a similar injury today probably would cost five or six times as much, thanks largely to sophisticated diagnostic and monitoring equipment and higher fees by specialist physicians.

I was unbelievably fortunate. The three-inch-long hole in my head was my only souvenir of my brain injury. I resumed normal development. By the age of four I could read and was even writing short letters.

Because I was lucky enough to recover fully, my head injury was a source more of curiosity than of problems while I was growing up. The barber I went to when I was in high school joked with me about the dent. To camouflage it, he left the hair on the sides a little longer than was normal for a fifties' flattop. Coaches and friends kidded me about those wings of hair flapping as I dribbled the basketball down the court.

For my mother and my grandmother, though, the emotional trauma was intense and enduring. Whenever barbers asked my mother about the hole in her little boy's head, explaining it to them brought back the anguish that she had felt the afternoon of the accident. For years afterward, she worried that I would have another head injury. She also fretted about the possibility that other small children, especially those under her care, would be seriously injured. When my own children were around two years old, my mother was seized by an irrational fear that she would have the same experience as her mother—that some horrible accident would happen to her grandchildren while she was responsible for them. Fortunately, history didn't repeat itself.

Of course, my grandmother was greatly relieved that I recovered fully. Later, she confided to my mother that if I hadn't survived, she wouldn't have been able to live with her guilt. She said that she would have taken her own life. I always felt a special bond with my grandmother; eventually I came to realize that our relationship was so meaningful and intimate partly because of my early brush with death.

Only years later, after learning much more about the suffering endured by the families of brain-injury victims, was I able to appreciate the emotional trauma and anxieties that my family experienced after my accident and during my recuperation. At least they met with a positive outcome at the end of their ordeal.

What I know about my brain injury, I've learned from conversations with my family and with Max Bernauer. Twenty-two years after my accident, I called Dr. Bernauer, who was then in his mid-seventies but still practicing medicine. At my request, he reviewed my medical records and met with me to discuss them. He confirmed that his sole treatment had been to remove bone fragments and place the shunt. He had left all else to time and the natural healing process.

"Nature is kind to little children," he told me. Later, neurosurgeon Richard Weiner and neuropsychologist Harvey Levin suggested that Dr. Bernauer was only partly right. Although children's brains, like the rest of their bodies, do heal faster than those of adults, the youngest head injury victims often face a lifetime of limitations. Infants and toddlers are especially likely to develop learning disabilities and post-traumatic epilepsy.

As a young adult, I was fascinated rather than embarrassed by the hole in my head and the remarkable episode that caused it. Once, while working as a volunteer in a local hospital, I asked the X-ray technician to take a picture of my skull. He did so, but the image wasn't particularly interesting. It revealed nothing new— only that my skull had been fractured and my brain bruised. That satisfied my curiosity, at least for a while. More recently, thanks to subsequent advances in technology, a computerized tomography (CT) scan done in 1985 showed cross sections of my brain with the

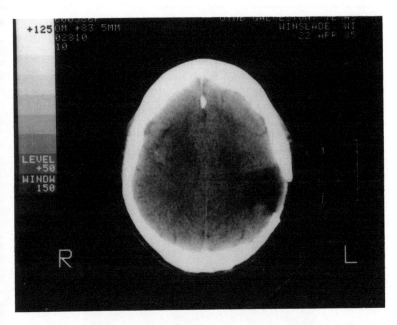

Figure 1. CT scan made in 1985. Courtesy of Richard Weiner, M.D.

portion of my skull missing (Figure 1). Later, a magnetic resonance image (MRI) revealed a white area indicating the fluid sac that had formed, somewhat like scar tissue, where my head had smashed against the concrete (Figure 2).

According to physicians who have reviewed that MRI, the extent to which my brain was damaged is unclear. Fortunately, the trauma didn't interfere with my physical or intellectual development.

Throughout my professional career, I've been fascinated by the human brain. Consciousness, reasoning, dreaming, memory, and all our other mental capacities have always struck me as remarkable. As an undergraduate, I first encountered Descartes and his declaration, "I think, therefore I am." Then and later, when I was studying for my doctorate in philosophy, I found the fact that we could think about thinking astonishing. When I subsequently

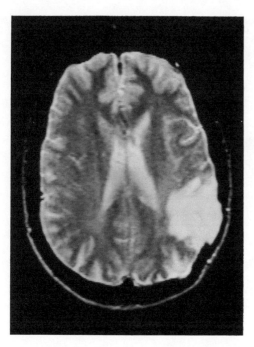

Figure 2. MRI *made in 1989 showing fluid sac at wound site.*
Courtesy of Melvyn Schreiber, M.D.

studied law, especially the issues of mental responsibility and insanity, I was struck by the legal puzzles raised when an individual's mental processes were disordered or dysfunctional. My work as a psychoanalyst focused my attention on yet other dimensions of brain activity—such intriguing psychological phenomena as unconscious desires, fantasies, and dreams.

My attention has most recently been consumed by two other issues involving the human brain. One is the maze of problems raised by the loss of consciousness, especially those concerning people who have become permanently unconscious. The second, which all too often intersects the first, is the subject of this book—traumatic brain injury as a major public health problem. In spite of the dramatic drop in brain trauma that began in the early 1960s, partly because of car safety devices like seat belts and, later, air bags—lifesaving devices long resisted by Detroit's auto makers as being too expensive—the rate of fatal brain trauma in the United States remains inexcusably high. Of every 100,000 Americans, up to 25 die every year from this single cause. This is twice the rate of such deaths in the United Kingdom, Sweden, or Japan. And the number who survive but suffer the disabling effects of traumatic brain injury is far higher. We need to examine its causes and its costs to patients, families, health professionals, and society as a whole. We must explore possible solutions to the problems it creates. And we have to take individual and collective action to reduce both the incidence and the consequences of brain trauma.

Despite my childhood accident, my professional interest in traumatic brain injury developed relatively late. Like many Americans, I was aware of such well-known head injury cases as those of former White House press secretary James Brady, struck in 1981 by a bullet intended for Ronald Reagan, and Nancy Cruzan, the young Missouri woman whose car wreck in 1983 plunged her into a persistent vegetative state and the courts into a quandary over a family's right to have life support removed. But the issue came home to me, quite literally, when my family and I moved to Texas from California.

Because real estate prices were so much lower in Galveston than they'd been in Los Angeles, we were able to buy a handsome, spacious contemporary house on the edge of a lagoon. I was delighted by the location and the view, but one feature of our new home puzzled me: when the previous owners, Robert L. "Bobby" Moody, Jr., and his wife, had converted the garage into a separate apartment, they'd modified the bathroom to accommodate someone in a wheelchair. Our real estate agent told me that the Moodys had a son, Russell, who had suffered a severe brain injury.

When the accident occurred, nineteen-year-old Russell Moody

had just completed his freshman year at the University of Texas at Austin. His grades were average, he excelled at track and football, and his social skills and sense of humor made him very popular. On the afternoon of June 2, 1980, Russell pulled out of a gas station on one of the busy streets leading to Galveston's beaches. Another vehicle rear-ended his Jeep, catapulting Russell 150 feet. He landed headfirst in a concrete parking lot. The impact shattered a massive portion of the right side of his skull and lacerated the surface of the gray matter just beneath. Bruising and other diffuse neuronal damage extended throughout his brain.

Fortunately, in less than forty-five minutes Russell reached the emergency room of John Sealy Hospital, part of the University of Texas Medical Branch (UTMB). An immediate CT scan assessed and located the damage, and a neurosurgeon operated quickly to remove bone fragments and dead brain tissue and to reduce intracranial pressure. Russell's doctors feared that despite their speedily administered, state-of-the-art efforts, his injuries might prove fatal, but he survived. In the weeks after his initial surgery, his care focused on the crucial tasks of controlling brain swelling and infection, keeping his airways clear of mucous, and feeding him through a tube. It was more than a month before Russell began to respond to commands. Even after three months, his responses were limited to eye blinks and movements of his left arm and hand, and his reactions remained minimal and intermittent well into the fall. Six months after the accident, the physical, occupational, and speech therapists noted that he could hold his head up, respond to directions appropriately and consistently, and use his fingers to answer questions—one finger for "yes," two for "no."

On January 5, 1981, Russell Moody moved to Del Oro Hospital, fifty miles away in Houston. In all, he was hospitalized for three years. Eventually, Russell's medical, physical, neurological, and psychosocial functioning began to improve, but no one could tell how much further he would progress. Bobby Moody was committed to helping his son regain as many of his previous capabilities as possible. Cost was no obstacle. The Moody family's fortune was one of the oldest and largest in Texas, having been founded in the nineteenth century on cotton, banking, and railroads and in the early twentieth century on insurance. But none of the rehabilitation programs in the Galveston-Houston area struck Bobby Moody as adequate for Russell, so the Moody Foundation established the Transitional Learning Community (TLC) for patients disabled by traumatic brain injuries. Since it opened in 1984, TLC has helped more than six hundred head-trauma victims by combining physical, speech, recreational, and occupational therapy with retraining in the practical skills necessary for independent living.

Russell spent three years at TLC. He credits his rehabilitation nurse, Sheridan Barnes, and his family, especially his father, with giving him the support and care he needed as he struggled to relearn the basic tasks of everyday life. The emotional volatility that often trails in the wake of serious head injury exacerbated his frustration with the tedious process of reeducation, but he came to terms with that. Gradually, Russell recovered his brain and cognitive function, despite continuing medical problems and permanent physical handicaps. The once-promising athlete must use two canes to walk, but his sense of humor is intact.

Fortunately for Russell, his family's support was enduring, their financial resources were extraordinary, and his personal motivation was high. Even after his ordeal of six years of recovery and rehabilitation and his acceptance of the mobility limitations that will always be with him, he remains surprisingly optimistic. Now, eighteen years after the injury that could have killed him, Russell has an independent life and is happily married. He has been able to achieve much more than anyone could have imagined in the days and months following his accident.

After learning about Russell, I told Bobby Moody that I was also a fortunate survivor of a traumatic brain injury, hastening to point out that my family and I had been spared the tremendous ordeals that Russell and his family had faced. In response to my interest, Mr. Moody gave me a videotape called *Broken Rhymes*. It documented the efforts of Russell and three other young men to overcome near-fatal brain injuries and to recapture their lives. At the time, I had no idea that millions of other people shared their plight.

The documentary awakened me to the scope and complexity of the problems surrounding traumatic brain injury. I discovered that many physicians, neuroscientists, nurses, psychologists, and social workers, as well as occupational, physical, linguistic, and other kinds of therapists, devoted their professional lives to studying and treating brain trauma.

Why, I wondered as I watched the documentary, is the problem so large? What can and should be done to help those who survive traumatic brain injuries? Since we know how to prevent most of them, why do so many continue to happen? My attempts to answer these basic questions led me to study the literature, talk to professionals in the head injury field, and become acquainted with survivors and their families. Although I had been touched personally by this silent epidemic, it became clear that I knew little about it. As I found out more, I began to realize that injuries like Russell's and mine were part of an overwhelming medical and public health problem.

Some reporting agencies still lumped traumatic brain injuries under their causes. For example, states often do a single tally of deaths or disabilities from vehicular accidents, without distinguishing which result from brain trauma and which from crushed chests or severed spinal cords. Because of this, absolute numbers for the devastating toll taken by brain trauma are hard to come by. Throughout this book, I have cited figures that, to my best judgment, are the most accurate available. By even the most conservative estimate, traumatic brain injury stands along with cardiovascular disease, cancer, and stroke as one of the major killers of the late twentieth century.

According to the Brain Injury Association, every year more than 2 million people in the United States suffer traumatic brain injuries, 373,000 of these severe enough to require hospitalization. Brain trauma is the leading cause of death among children and young adults. It kills at least 60,000 Americans annually and leaves 2,000 in a persistent vegetative state, unaware of their surroundings, unable to respond to even the most basic stimuli, and totally dependent on others. The March 1996 *Journal of Trauma* reported that 90,000 brain-injury victims require extended rehabilitation each year. Many if not most such victims endure lifelong physical, mental, and emotional impairments ranging from blurred vision to paralysis, from memory problems to poor judgment, from fatigue to inappropriate behavior in social situations. More than half of all victims of severe head trauma are young men from fifteen to twenty-four years of age; all too often, their brain injuries rob them and the rest of us of their entire productive adulthood. Survivors of a severe brain injury typically face five to ten years of intensive rehabilitation aimed at helping them recover enough of their capacities to live independent, if limited, lives. Over an individual's lifetime, the expense of brain trauma can exceed $4 million. When the costs of treatment and rehabilitation are combined, the nation's annual bill for traumatic brain injury amounts to $4.8 billion, according to the Brain Injury Association. Lost productivity undoubtedly would add several billions more to that staggering total.

Scientists have yet to understand exactly how brain injury affects thought, memory, speech, movement, and behavior, but *how* most brain traumas occur is no mystery. More than half result from vehicular mishaps—car, truck, motorcycle, and bike accidents. Assaults (especially gunshot wounds), falls, suicides and attempted suicides, and sports injuries account for most of the rest. Tragically, 64 percent of children under the age of one who are abused sustain brain injury, according to the Brain Injury Association. Moreover, the association calculates that close to thirty thousand children each year develop permanent disabilities as a consequence of traumatic brain injuries.

Thousands of professionals and millions of survivors know firsthand the complex medical, social, psychological, and ethical issues raised by traumatic brain injury. For them the epidemic isn't silent; it's nearly deafening. Yet as I continued my research, I realized that the general public is only dimly aware of traumatic brain injury. Combating the brain-trauma crisis demands a collective effort because the problems it raises are public problems. Not only do they challenge our medical, scientific, and technical capabilities; they stress our economy, our political and legal systems, and our cultural assumptions as well. Addressing the problems born of traumatic brain injury will require reordering social priorities and confronting tenaciously held attitudes, beliefs, and values.

First, we must recognize that when it comes to injury in general and traumatic brain injury in particular, the problems that we as a society share are growing at an alarming rate. Thanks to advances in trauma care, our ability to save lives far outstrips our ability to restore function to victims of serious brain trauma. Those who survive with severe disabilities require decades of chronic care at catastrophic costs. Even survivors with good insurance soon reach the maximum coverage. Then, unless the family ranks among the rare few with wealth in the millions, the cost of such care quickly exhausts its resources. Once that happens, Medicaid takes over, and we all pay the bill.

As a bioethicist trained in both philosophy and the law and intensely interested in fairness, I am particularly concerned that people with traumatic brain injuries receive appropriate treatment. Typically, as the cases and statistics presented here show, the quality, quantity, and duration of rehabilitative care depend on what financial resources are available rather than on what will most benefit a victim of traumatic brain injury. While their insurance lasts, patients with little hope of recovery often receive expensive services developed for patients with a better prognosis; meanwhile, uninsured patients are denied this same help, even when it could make the difference between a life of dependency and one of relatively full function. Clearly, our society is neither efficiently nor effectively serving the needs of people who have suffered serious brain trauma.

Of course, we can do the most good by preventing severe head injuries in the first place. The amount of traumatic brain injury currently tolerated in our society is inexcusable. Everyone acknowledges that prevention is important, and the limited steps that we've taken have proven effective. For example, motorcycle and bicycle helmets significantly reduce the incidence of traumatic brain injury. We know other measures that would cut the staggering traumatic brain injury statistics. But we must act — through public policy and individual conduct.

In the long run, our goal must be to diminish violence and reckless risk taking and to encourage civility and concern for others. To accomplish this transformation, I believe, we should prefer rational positive and negative incentives, such as insurance discounts and penalties, over moralistic or punitive measures. I harbor no illusions that rational persuasion alone can prevent violent or reckless behavior, but sustained, systematic public education will be necessary, even though it may not be sufficient.

Traumatic brain injury can be reduced. But needless deaths and tremendous suffering can be prevented only if we make halting this silent epidemic a priority. That will take innovative policies, political courage, government support, financial commitment, widespread education, and individual willingness to change—in short, a collective paradigm shift in our values accompanied by action. We must alter both our attitudes and our behavior. If we don't, the costs—economic and emotional—will drive us not just to bankruptcy but to despair.

· o n e ·

Our Vulnerable Brains

During World War II, a Russian soldier named Leva Zazetsky suffered a wound from a bullet that penetrated his skull and severely
damaged his brain. For the rest of his life, he experienced the world
in a bizarrely fragmented way. Although he appeared to be normal,
he could remember neither the names of objects nor the meanings of words. Although he could talk, when he tried to speak he
couldn't find the words to communicate his ideas and feelings. Before the war he had been a fourth-year student at a technical university; after his injury he couldn't read or perform simple addition.

The unfortunate young man's sense of space and his physical
orientation to the world were severely disrupted. He could see only
out of the left sides of both eyes. He simply had no visual awareness
of things on the right side of his field of vision. He would see only
parts of objects or sometimes not see them at all. For example, if he
had a bowl of soup in front of him, he might be able to see merely
a bit of the spoon, or he even might lose the spoon entirely if it was

on his right side. In addition to leaving him able to see only parts of objects, Zazetsky's brain injury also caused him to have hallucinations. Ugly faces and rooms with odd shapes would appear when he closed his eyes, so he would open them immediately. This made it very difficult for him to sleep.

Neuropsychologist A. R. Luria worked with Zazetsky as he struggled valiantly to piece back together his disintegrated life. For twenty-five years, Zazetsky kept a journal, using it to try to recapture the thoughts, experiences, feelings, and memories that had been ripped away by the bullet that tore into his brain. In *The Man with the Shattered World: The History of a Brain Wound,* a book first published in Russian in 1972, Dr. Luria explained: "His only material consisted of fragmentary recollections that came to mind at random. On these he had to impose some order and sense of continuity though every word he recalled, every thought he expressed required the most excruciating effort. When his writing went well he managed to write a page a day, two at the most, and felt completely drained with this. Writing was his only link with life, his only hope of not succumbing to illness but recovering at least a part of what had been lost. This journal recounts a desperate fight for life with a skill psychologists cannot help but envy."

Dr. Luria tried to comprehend as a neuropsychologist what Zazetsky described as an existential trauma. At their first meeting, three months after the bullet wound, Zazetsky couldn't recall what had happened at the battlefront where he was injured. Finally, he remembered that it was the month of May. Then he was able to retrieve the names of the other months, but he couldn't remember, for example, which month came before September, and he couldn't remember the seasons.

Although he could see, Zazetsky couldn't interpret the things he saw. In order to learn how to read again, first he had to relearn the meanings of letters. Because he saw the visual world in shattered

fragments, he could read only a few letters at a time. He had to retain these as he moved across the page, picking up other letters to
combine into a single word.

Writing was easier, especially after Zazetsky realized that he could
write quickly and automatically, getting a whole word down without thinking about the letters that made it up. Apparently the
part of his brain that allowed him to write hadn't been destroyed.
Eventually he could write as well as he had before his injury, even
though he remained unable to read what he had put on the page.

Zazetsky's confusion about spatial relationships caused him to
get lost even a short distance from his house and made him unable
to comprehend directions. He didn't recognize places with which
he'd been very familiar before his injury. In his journal, Zazetsky
described how his visual problems and lack of spatial orientation
would cause him to lose track of whole parts of his body: "Often
I fall into a kind of stupor and don't understand what's going on
around me. I have no sense of objects. One minute I stand there
thinking about something; the next I lapse into forgetfulness. But
suddenly I'll come to look at the right of me and be horrified to discover half my body is gone. I'm terrified. I try to figure out what's
become of my right arm and leg, the entire right side of my body. I
move the fingers of my left hand, feel them, but can't see the fingers
of my right hand, and somehow I'm not even aware they're there."

The details of Zazetsky's story are unusual. Certainly his determination and persistence are rare. But medical history is replete
with cases in which traumatic brain injuries have robbed their victims of some mental faculties but not others, and there is a simple
reason for this: different parts of the brain coordinate different
functions.

The astonishing three-pound organ responsible for both our
basic, animal survival and for all aspects of our personality and personal identity is fragile. Cars, bullets, fists, baseballs, and horses'

hooves can damage it; indirectly, so can gravity—when we fall or when something falls on us. And because we live in a world filled with such hazards, we are all vulnerable. Who hasn't bumped his or her head or been hit in the head by some projectile? Maybe the bump caused only a momentary pain, or perhaps a tender swelling formed. If the blow was hard enough, it may have been followed by nausea or dizziness. Being smacked by something soft like a beach ball causes no harm, but if a baseball fouled into stands collides with a human head at forty miles per hour, it can mean serious injury.

Because traumatic brain injury has always been part of the human experience, healers have puzzled over the brain's workings since prehistory. "Head injuries must have been very common in the life of primitive people, given the harsh and dangerous conditions of their existence," neuropsychologist Harvey Levin observes, "and they must have been quite familiar with some of the consequences of these injuries." In the oldest known medical document, the Edwin Smith Surgical Papyrus, itself a copy of an older manuscript written about 3000 B.C., ancient Egyptians noted a correlation between left-side skull fractures and paralysis or loss of speech.

Surgical repair of traumatic brain injuries also dates back for millennia. Physicians in ancient Greece developed instruments for removing bone fragments from depressed skull fractures and for cutting holes in the skull to repair head wounds. As the centuries passed, surgical techniques evolved for treating skull fractures, intracranial pressure and swelling of the brain, and arrow, spear, and gunshot wounds.

Since Plato and Aristotle, philosophers have scrutinized the nature of human consciousness, thought, and reason. In the seventeenth century, the French philosopher René Descartes was preoccupied with the unique consciousness of self that seems to set us apart from other creatures. He also cleared the path for future research on how the brain functions by a style of analysis that threw out old dogmas and reduced complex concepts to their simplest components and by regarding the human brain and body as machinery. As his successors struggled to describe, classify, and explain consciousness, they established the branches of philosophy called philosophy of mind and epistemology, which together later spawned psychology.

Long before scientific evidence made the connection clear, astute observers began associating consciousness with brain functions. The ancient Greek physician Hippocrates suspected that the brain was the source of awareness, thought, and feeling. Apart from his followers, few agreed. For centuries, the heart, spleen, and liver were considered more essential to human identity than the brain.

Modern brain research began in the nineteenth century. Although Sigmund Freud is best known for his work on dreams, suppressed desires, language, and reactions to emotional trauma, his earliest theory concerned a biology of the mind. Like other scientists of his day, he believed that human psychology ultimately rested upon the complexities of the brain.

Half a century earlier, in 1837, Marc Dax, a French physician who was examining patients who had lost the ability to speak, noticed a link to paralysis on the right side of the body and injury to the left side of the brain. During an autopsy of a stroke victim who could utter but a single word, Parisian surgeon Paul Broca discovered that the only part of the man's brain that was damaged was a specific area called the posterior frontal cortex. Later he checked out eight other patients' similarly impaired speech and found that seven of them had suffered damage to the very same region. Subsequent research sought to map the parts of the brain that controlled various functions—sight, consciousness, memory, learning, language, and even moral sense. The concept known as "localization" was now firmly established.

One case that drew considerable attention was that of Phineas Gage. In 1848, Gage was a twenty-five-year-old construction foreman for the Rutland and Burlington Railroad. His job included supervising the setting of explosives for leveling the Vermont terrain so that the work crew could lay track. Typically, an assistant drilled a hole in the rock, filled it with blasting powder, and covered it with sand. Then Gage would tamp it all down with a three-centimeter-thick iron rod and set the fuse. One September day, something distracted Gage, and he tamped the powder directly—before his assistant could pour in the sand. In the resulting explosion, the rod went straight through Gage's skull and brain, entering the left side of his face and exiting above his forehead.

Remarkably, with some assistance, Gage was able to walk away from the accident. Although he was stunned, he never lost consciousness or the ability to speak clearly. His left eye was gone, but otherwise he recovered completely.

Except for one thing: before the accident, Phineas Gage had been an exceptionally responsible young man who behaved in accordance with the strict social conventions of his day. After his traumatic brain injury, he became unreliable and irreverent. He peppered his speech with profanities, and he couldn't hold a job. When Gage died in 1861, no autopsy was performed, but twenty years later a scientist named John Harlow retrieved his skull, examined it, and posited that the key to responsible and appropriate behavior lay somewhere in the left frontal lobe of the brain—the portion devastated in Gage's accident.

The recognition that specific areas of the brain direct specific functions helps to explain why the unfortunate Zazetsky could write more easily than he could read, why he could view the left side of his body but not the right, and why he could display normal intelligence in some activities but couldn't find his way home from a few blocks away.

In her book *The Broken Brain,* psychiatrist Nancy C. Andreasen describes the brain as composed of tissue with the consistency of Jell-O. It floats inside the skull, encased in a protective sac, which is called the *dura mater,* and cushioned by cerebrospinal fluid. The brain's gray surface is a maze of ridges; beneath them, most of the brain is white. Its curious appearance gives few clues to how it operates.

Viewed from the top, the brain is arranged in two hemispheres, left and right. The large mass extending from the forehead to the back of the skull is the cerebrum, the part that directs language, learning, creativity, introspection, and all the higher functions that we think of as giving us a human existence. Scientists subdivide each hemisphere of the cerebrum into four lobes (Figure 3). Farthest to the back, the occipital lobe takes in and disseminates visual information. Jutting out to the side, the temporal lobe handles hearing, language, and memory. Immediately above these two, the parietal lobe deals with other sensory data and regulates spatial orientation. The cerebrum's frontal lobe is the least understood part of the brain. Part of it controls our movements; other parts are devoted to different aspects of thinking, feeling, and decision making.

Immediately under the cerebrum lie the diencephalon, the basal ganglia, and the pituitary, the tiny gland that regulates hormones. Within the diencephalon, the thalamus modulates emotions, sensations, and behavior, serving as a sort of switching center between the cerebrum and the body, while the hypothalamus oversees hormonal function. Working with the cerebellum, which is located at the base of the skull, the basal ganglia control movement. Hidden beneath the cerebellum is the most primitive part of the brain — the midbrain, pons, and finally the medulla, which connects directly to the spinal cord. Often referred to collectively as the brain

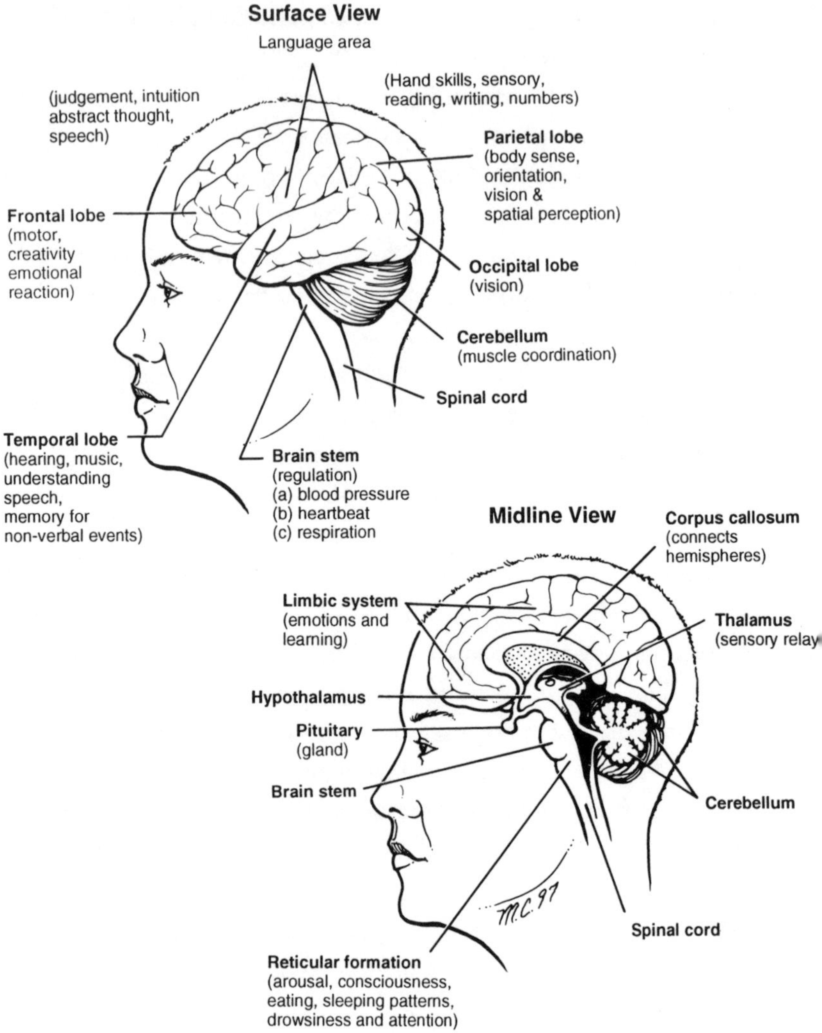

Surface View

Language area

(judgement, intuition abstract thought, speech)

(Hand skills, sensory, reading, writing, numbers)

Parietal lobe
(body sense, orientation, vision & spatial perception)

Frontal lobe
(motor, creativity emotional reaction)

Occipital lobe
(vision)

Cerebellum
(muscle coordination)

Spinal cord

Temporal lobe
(hearing, music, understanding speech, memory for non-verbal events)

Brain stem
(regulation)
(a) blood pressure
(b) heartbeat
(c) respiration

Midline View

Corpus callosum
(connects hemispheres)

Limbic system
(emotions and learning)

Thalamus
(sensory relay)

Hypothalamus

Pituitary
(gland)

Brain stem

Cerebellum

Spinal cord

Reticular formation
(arousal, consciousness, eating, sleeping patterns, drowsiness and attention)

Figure 3. The human brain. Drawing by Michael Cooley.

stem, these structures are responsible for heartbeat, respiration, and other vital functions—in other words, for the most basic aspects of organic survival.

Whatever its function, each part of the brain is made up primarily of nerve cells. These come in two types: neurons, which do the work, and glial cells, which support and nourish the neurons. Neurons communicate with each other through axons—thin tubes that run like microscopic wires through the brain, carrying electrical messages. Axons serve as transmission lines for signals to and from the brain and between its various parts. When the head accelerates, stops, or twists violently, these delicate fibers can stretch, tear, or shear off. Such axonal damage can prevent sensory information from reaching the brain and keep the brain's commands from getting back to the limbs. On a smaller scale, it can interrupt the internal signals essential for the brain itself to function normally.

Scientists have yet to unravel how the brain's individual structures do what they do, let alone how they interact with one another. Some neurophysiologists look at the brain as a biochemical system; others see it as a complex web of electrical circuits similar to those of a computer. Like the nineteenth-century view of the brain as a machine, each of these models can be useful, but none tells the whole story of this complex organic system. Dr. Andreasen notes that the brain's "designer, if it had one, concealed it well from hostile forces, in addition to concealing well its organization and function." She goes on to describe one of the most helpful metaphors: the brain as a network of scattered information centers that use electrical impulses to communicate among themselves: "Different areas of gray matter are specialized in different functions, such as moving, seeing, touching, listening, thinking, or modulating physical functions such as eating or sleeping. Often these areas are redundant—that is, several areas can perform the same function.

Thus, when one communication center is knocked out, another may be able to take over in its place."

Another of Dr. Andreasen's insights is crucial to understanding traumatic brain injury. Inside its bony case, its tough *dura mater,* and its cushion of fluid, "the brain itself is soft, delicate, and easily damaged. If you touch it too hard, it may bleed."

Although many blows to the head are inconsequential, some have significant, if not permanently disabling, effects. For example, while my younger daughter, Marcia, was doing a flip during gymnastics practice, she landed on her head. She had headaches for weeks afterward. Fortunately, they eventually ceased. A few years ago, my older daughter, Joanna, was hit on the head by a fifty-pound barbell while she was exercising before swimming practice. At first, she denied that the blow had caused any harm, but soon a large swelling arose. Then she experienced double vision and a severe headache. To our great relief, a visit to the emergency room followed by a CT scan revealed no serious damage.

Joanna was lucky. One of my former colleagues at UCLA was in a traffic accident and smashed her head on her car's windshield. Medical examinations revealed no injury to her skull, and various kinds of high-tech imaging showed no visible damage to her brain. Yet for months afterward she couldn't think clearly or concentrate, nor could she keep track of multiple intellectual tasks. She found this particularly frustrating in her job as a high-level university administrator.

At first, my colleague denied the problems. Some of her associates thought she might be malingering. Eventually, however, a neurologist explained that so-called minor brain injuries like hers —those not visibly discernible even through high-tech diagnostic procedures—can cause symptoms serious enough to disrupt the victims' lives, at least temporarily. In time, these symptoms often diminish or disappear, but meanwhile, the neurologist advised, my colleague would have to compensate by reducing the number of tasks that she undertook simultaneously or keeping careful lists to remind her of what she should do next.

Many things can damage the brain. Tumors, strokes, drug and alcohol overdoses, fever, and Parkinson's disease all kill brain cells; so do cardiovascular and respiratory disorders or anything else that deprives those cells of oxygen. But my focus here is brain damage that results when the head is hit, is penetrated, strikes a stationary object, or is violently shaken or twisted. Unlike brain damage caused by chemicals or disease or the failure of some other body system, such as the lungs or heart, traumatic brain injury occurs suddenly and immediately produces varying and often multiple functional deficits. With the possible exception of chemical insults, traumatic brain injury is the most preventable cause of brain damage. Because of this, and because so many of its victims are young and therefore face decades of disability, brain trauma is also the most crucial for us to examine as a society.

Traumatic brain injuries fall into two basic categories: penetrating and closed. Penetrating wounds often look the most serious. The sight of someone with a sharp object sticking out of his or her head is among the most horrifying imaginable. Yet, depending on the missile's speed and trajectory, on the exact areas of the brain it damaged, and on many things that scientists have yet to discover, such wounds can result in anything from death to little or no impairment. Phineas Gage walked away, dazed but talking, after having an iron rod shoot through his skull; Zazetsky spent his life struggling to integrate his shattered world after a much smaller bullet entered his brain; President John Kennedy died a few hours after a gunshot wound to the head.

Amazing as they may seem, penetrating head injuries with few lasting effects are not as rare as the often bizarre particulars of individual cases might lead us to believe. Provided that infection is prevented, the brain breached by a sharp object can sometimes re-organize itself, circumventing the injured portion.

Consider the man who was admitted in a drunken stupor to the emergency room of Massachusetts General Hospital. He suffered from a slight limp, and the right side of his face drooped. Other than that, nothing much seemed wrong with him once he sobered up. But a CT scan taken while he was still semiconscious revealed the clear image of a three-inch nail inside his brain, its point touching the back of his skull. Asked how it got there, the patient explained that twelve years earlier he had tried to commit suicide by shooting himself between the eyes with a nail gun.

Closed head injuries, on the other hand, may look less serious on superficial inspection but may cause far more harm. Ironically, that's because the bony case that protects the brain also can damage it. The inside of the human skull is a mass of hard ridges. During normal movements, such as nods or rotations, and even light impacts, these ridges help keep the brain floating in place. But because the skull, the cerebrospinal fluid, and the brain all have different densities, when the head accelerates suddenly, as it does when a boxer takes an uppercut to the jaw, or decelerates quickly, as it did when my colleague's head hit her windshield, these three don't move at the same speed. This makes the brain bounce around against the hard, rough surface of the skull, causing abrasions and bruising that can extend all the way to the brain stem. Violent twisting and vibration can produce similar diffuse damage, which is why shaking a child—especially a very young one—is a potentially disastrous form of discipline.

The elderly have their own special vulnerabilities to head injury. Owing to osteoporosis and problems with balance, the latter often exacerbated by alcohol and prescription drugs, people over sixty-five suffer a disproportionate number of falls, and because their reflexes have slowed, they have trouble protecting their heads as they tumble. Moreover, our brains shrink as we age, leaving more space for the brain to travel inside the skull; a bump on the head that would barely faze a twenty-five-year-old may cause his or her grandfather lasting damage.

Blows to the head are among the most common causes of closed brain injury. Rocks, clubs, baseballs, and countless other hard objects, whether dropped, thrown, or wielded, are capable of shattering the skull without breaking the skin. The potential sources of damage vary from place to place (for example, falling coconuts cause many head injuries in Micronesia but few in the continental United States), but the results are similar. A single sharp thump can produce several types of immediate damage. If blunt trauma crushes the skull, bone fragments may bruise, cut, or penetrate the brain, causing injury. If the impact comes from the side, rotating the head suddenly, nerve fibers and blood vessels can be torn.

Among the most devastating effects of head injury is the secondary damage that can follow hours and days later. Like other parts of the body, the brain responds to bruising by swelling. But unlike the skin-covered leg or wrist, the bruised brain has nowhere to go once it reaches the inelastic skull. When this happens, pressure builds, and arteries and veins can be squeezed so tight that circulation to the bruised portion of the brain shuts down. The resulting oxygen deprivation can cause death or irreversible damage. Blood leaking from a wound inside the skull can form clots, or hematomas, that compress the area of the brain beneath them. The fluid that collects as a reaction to the initial injury can cause hydrocephalus. Draining it off lowers the intracranial pressure that may cause more devastation than the original impact. The higher the intracranial pressure and the longer it lasts, the more irreversible damage the brain suffers. That is why closed head wounds often wreak more havoc than nastier-looking penetrating wounds, which provide their own drains. (And that is why the shunt that

Dr. Bernauer inserted in my skull and the speed with which he placed it were essential to my recovery.)

Scientists still don't understand how the brain heals itself, so long-term recovery from any traumatic brain injury is uncertain, and its course is difficult to predict. Some victims recover spontaneously. Until recently, neuroscientists thought that much of the loss of capabilities due to brain damage was irreversible. We now know that rehabilitation sometimes can restore cognitive and functional skills and emotional and experiential capacity, at least in part. Physical, occupational, recreational, and educational therapies may have significant short- or long-term benefits in certain cases. Although a good deal of rigorous evaluation must take place before we will know which of the various therapies currently available or under development will work in which kinds of cases, preliminary research suggests that for many victims of traumatic brain injury, the potential for recovery is much greater than previously believed.

Recovery from traumatic brain injury may be quick or slow; it may be complete, partial, or absent. It may come easily or require immense and intense effort. The anguish felt by the patient and his or her family may give way at last to success, or their hopes may end in despair.

People who do recover from traumatic brain injury must be highly motivated and persistent. Supportive families, skilled therapists, and protective environments in which to relearn the tasks of living and make the transition from hospital to outside world play an essential role. Treatment and other resources must be available and affordable, but a certain amount of physiological luck also comes into play. So does a constellation of factors and forces that currently lies beyond the reach of science yet cannot be fully explained by faith and hope.

The most comforting stories about recovery from traumatic brain injury have the timeless power of great myths. We love both the tales of miraculous escape, like Phineas Gage's, and the epics of valiant persistence and strength of character, like Russell Moody's. But we should not let these individual accounts obscure the fact that the broad spectrum of outcomes goes from full recovery to death, with a range of disabilities, many of them horrendous, in between. As we formulate our public policies and conduct our own lives, we must bear in mind that many individuals with traumatic brain injury never recover enough to lead independent lives. Their need for chronic care poses haunting challenges to our society.

· t w o ·

Saving Lives: The Golden Hour

Emergency room doctors and nurses speak of the "golden hour." If the victim's airways are open and he or she isn't hemorrhaging from a major artery, then the body's vital systems continue to function relatively well for about sixty minutes following major trauma. After that, those systems left unaided tend to decline toward death or permanent damage to major organs. Treatment of severe traumatic brain injury almost always involves surgery, and the patient wheeled into the operating room within or close to that golden hour stands a much better chance of surviving the stress of an operation. If surgery isn't performed within four hours, a victim of a serious closed head injury usually is beyond saving. One San Diego study followed eighty-two brain-trauma patients with subdural hematomas—blood clots under the brain's tough outer layer. The mortality rate was 30 percent for those operated on within four hours of injury, 90 percent for those who waited longer.

In severe head trauma, it's not just the sudden mechanical damage that kills and disables. Much of the destruction results from what neuroscientists call secondary insults. Many of these delayed injuries result from the brain's reaction to the initial impact. Take the most immediately life-threatening secondary insult, lack of oxygen. Although accounting for only one-fiftieth of the body's weight, the brain demands one-fifth of its oxygen. Without oxygen, brain cells begin to die within six minutes. A fall or motorcycle accident may block a victim's airway or cause bleeding severe enough to interrupt the flow of oxygen to the brain. Or hematomas pressing on sections of the brain can cut off the supply to those areas. Such clots are the major cause of what neuroscientists call "talk-and-die syndrome," in which a patient is conscious and oriented enough to speak after a head injury yet doesn't survive.

Like any bruised or lacerated tissue, the battered brain swells. But unlike an injured muscle, the swollen brain can expand only so far. When it reaches the bony casing of the skull, the internal pressure builds, squeezing blood vessels and cutting off the flow of oxygen and nutrients. Half of all brain-injury deaths in patients who reach the hospital alive result from this uncontrolled pressure.

Even when the seriously injured brain gets enough oxygen, its chemical balance goes haywire. For reasons that medical science has yet to fathom, the injured brain becomes more acidic; until its pH, or acid-base balance, is brought under control, the whole brain, not just the injured part, operates abnormally. Because the brain regulates all physical functions essential to life, the victim may die or suffer permanent physical damage if the problem is not corrected quickly.

Ensuring such swift treatment is the job of, among others, Life Flight pilot Al Vaiani. He spends most of his workdays in John Sealy Hospital's trauma area—the part of the emergency room set aside for victims of life-threatening injuries. The physicians, nurses, and emergency medical technicians (EMTs) who work in the crash unit focus their skill and energy on two things: saving lives and preventing further damage during the crucial first few hours after injury. When a victim of accident or violence rolls through those doors, the trauma team puts on what basketball players would call a full court press.

From his small office, Vaiani supervises the care of the Life Flight helicopter, a specially equipped Messerschmidt BK-117 that he flies for the University of Texas Medical Branch. He also waits for codes to appear on his beeper's digital display: 1111 means "Stand by"; 1188, "Come on ahead."

Around the country, major medical centers retain services like Life Flight as the front line in their battle to save the lives of trauma victims. Trips from accident scene to emergency room that might take hours in an ambulance can be accomplished in minutes by air. Medical evacuation helicopters are nimble enough to land on railroad tracks. They fly loaded with essential drugs and equipment and staffed by emergency medical technicians (often registered nurses) trained in trauma care, so life-saving measures that once had to wait for the hospital can be performed at the scene and in flight.

Police, sheriff's deputies, state troopers, and fire departments' emergency medical service teams call on Life Flight to transport the victims of potentially fatal catastrophes ranging from heart attacks to knifings. But the most common are motor vehicle accidents, which are also the most frequent cause of severe head trauma: in the United States, 44 percent of traumatic brain injuries and 57 percent of head-injury deaths result from car, truck, van, and motorcycle wrecks. In about 70 percent of fatal vehicle crashes, brain trauma is the cause of death; in more than two-thirds of the automobile accidents in which people are hurt, someone suffers a head injury. The next most common culprit in brain trauma is violence, including gunshot wounds, accounting for 30 percent of cases. Serious falls, like my own plunge just before I turned two, are third, causing 10 percent of traumatic brain injury among the population in general and a larger proportion among young children and the elderly.

Head injury alone is sufficient reason for transport by Life Flight. That's because the speed with which a victim receives help often means the difference between life and death or between recovery and lifelong disability. Sixty percent of the people who die from brain trauma do so before reaching the hospital, and many of those expire because they just don't get there fast enough.

Because speed is so essential in trauma care, Al Vaiani's helicopter sits on a concrete pad just outside the John Sealy Hospital crash unit. Normally, he and the Life Flight team of two registered nurses, both trained in trauma care, lift off three and a half to five minutes after the 1188 code appears on his beeper. The nurses ride in the rear of the aircraft, which is fitted with two removable rigid backboards and hookups for the monitors and equipment that will help keep the victim or victims alive on the trip back. On the seat to Vaiani's right, a rack holds detailed maps to help him locate the scene of the injury. If the victim is lucky, the accident happens somewhere in the fifty miles between Galveston and Houston. Both cities have major medical centers staffed with neurosurgeons and equipped with the latest diagnostic technologies. And both have Life Flight helicopters. Vaiani can reach Friendswood, halfway to Houston, in twelve minutes.

Once he's airborne, Vaiani radios ahead to the police or troopers on the ground. He gets an update on the circumstances of the trauma, the number of victims, their conditions, and the characteristics of the site. If the victim crashed a car on the interstate, Vaiani asks for reassurance that traffic has been blocked off; if the victim drove it into a marsh, Vaiani needs to know the nearest dry place to land. He checks the location of any spilled fuel or downed power lines. If the head injury resulted from domestic violence or a drive-by shooting, Vaiani makes sure that police have secured the scene so he won't come under fire as he sets the craft down.

With the crew keeping an eye out for obstacles and for other aircraft, Vaiani lands on a hard surface 100 to 150 feet from the site. The nurses jump out, carrying a backboard piled with the equipment and medications that they think they'll need. Among these are an intravenous solution of mannitol, a diuretic drug that helps control brain swelling; a ten-inch cube that monitors blood pressure, heart rate, oxygen saturation, and carbon dioxide levels; both nasal and oral breathing tubes; and an ambu-bag, an oxygen unit fitted with a bag-valve mask.

Toting this potentially life-saving burden, the nurses walk briskly to the trauma scene. Sometimes the victim is still pinned in the wreckage. In that case, one of the trauma staff climbs in with him or her and gets to work while the Jaws of Life are cutting away at the metal.

The first step is to make sure that the victim is getting the oxygen the brain needs. That means seeing to it that the patient has an open airway and is breathing well enough on his or her own. "Oxygen is the one drug that you never withhold," explains trauma nurse Barbara Bowers, the program coordinator for Life Flight at the University of Texas Medical Branch. "If the patient is awake and alert, we give him the breather mask. If he's unconscious or real groggy, we intubate him."

Intubation is the process of inserting a flexible plastic breathing tube to open the victim's airway and prevent the tongue and mucous from blocking it. If the head injuries don't involve the face, nurses use nasal tubes; if the area around the nose is damaged, they use a mouth tube. In either case, they avoid tilting the victim's head back; if the patient has a crushed vertebra high in the neck, that could damage the spinal cord. Anyone suffering head trauma from a vehicle accident or a fall is likely to have other serious injuries as well. Once the patient is breathing, the trauma team immobilizes the head with a cervical collar and a head brace secured by one tape across the forehead and one across the chin. Then they treat any life-threatening bleeding or shock.

Stabilizing the victim well enough for transport takes no more than fifteen or twenty minutes. While they're working flat-out to get the patient to the hospital alive, the nurses try to assess the extent of the brain injury. They use a test called the Glasgow Coma Scale (see the accompanying table). The possible score ranges from three to fifteen points. A score of eight or fewer points indicates a serious brain injury; a reading of thirteen to fifteen generally points to relatively mild damage and a good chance of full recovery. But an alert accident victim can slip into unconsciousness, an initially comatose patient can begin to come around, and the alcohol intoxication common in both motor vehicle wrecks and falls can make a head injury seem more severe than it is. For these reasons, the nurses often perform the Glasgow twice—once on the scene and again en route—to detect changes for better or worse.

On the flight back to the hospital, the Life Flight staff monitors vital signs and gives the victim whatever help he or she needs to get to the emergency room with the best chance of survival and recovery. That often means starting intravenous mannitol and sometimes other drugs to reduce pressure inside the skull. It always means administering pure oxygen and monitoring the carbon dioxide level; keeping the amount of carbon dioxide below normal helps reduce brain swelling.

When the Life Flight helicopter touches down outside the trauma center, the crew unloads "hot"—with the helicopter's rotors still whirling—if they think the two and a half minutes required to shut them down will make a difference. The trauma staff rushes to stabilize the victim well enough to make it through

Glasgow Coma Scale

	Examiner's test	Patient's response	Assigned score
Eye opening	Spontaneous	Opens eyes on own	4
	Commands	Opens eyes when loudly asked to do so	3
	Pain	Opens eyes upon pressure	2
	Pain	Does not open eyes	1
Best motor response	Commands	Follows simple commands	6
	Pain	Pulls examiner's hand away upon pressure	5
	Pain	Pulls part of body away upon pressure	4
	Pain	Flexes body inappropriately to pain (decorticate posturing)	3
	Pain	Body becomes rigid in an extended position upon pressure (decerebrate posturing)	2
	Pain	Has no motor response to pressure	1
Verbal response	Speech	Carries on a lucid conversation and tells examiner where he or she is, who he or she is, and the month and year	5
	Speech	Seems confused or disoriented	4
	Speech	Says words that examiner can understand but makes no sense	3
	Speech	Makes sounds that examiner cannot understand	2
	Speech	Makes no sound	1

evaluation and surgery. With a helicopter evacuation patient, this generally takes no more than a few minutes; much of what the hospital trauma unit would do initially has already been done at the scene and in transit.

Until a few years ago, head injury victims went straight from the trauma unit to the operating room. Nowadays, they have a CT scan first. Invented in 1973, computerized tomography combines X rays with computer imaging to produce three-dimensional representations of the brain, visually slicing it into cross sections to pinpoint the operable lesions and hematomas caused by the head injury. A CT scan acts like radar, showing the brain surgeon where to cut. "If you operate without a CT scan, you might get into trouble," explains Greeley, Colorado, neurosurgeon Pam Harmann. "It's not the case, like you see in the movies, that external signs like a blown pupil on one side or paralysis on the other can tell you where the patient might have an operable lesion."

Sometimes the evaluation staff also uses magnetic resonance imaging, or MRI, which can pick up small lesions that CT scans may miss. "If there's an identifiable lesion, we'll operate on anyone who has any sign of life," Dr. Harmann says. An even more recent noninvasive imaging technique, positron emission tomography (PET), identifies irregularities in the brain's chemical balance and metabolism.

Even if no lesions or hematomas show up on scans, the brain may be seriously damaged. Life-threatening swelling can result from diffuse axonal injuries—the little bleedings that commonly occur when the head speeds up and then stops suddenly, as in vehicle accidents and falls. All too often, patients with traumatic brain injuries but normal CT scans end up dead, vegetative, or severely disabled. To prevent this, neurosurgeons frequently place a fiber-optic intracranial pressure monitor in one of the brain's fluid spaces, or ventricles, and a ventriculostomy to drain off excess fluid into a bag.

Surgery for severe head injury is an ordeal demanding hours of precise work on tiny structures within the restrictive confines of the skull. On March 31, 1981, when a bullet intended for Ronald Reagan hit his press secretary, James Brady, in the forehead, neurosurgeons needed six and a half hours to remove the trail of metal and bone fragments and the slug itself, which had lodged near his right ear. Brady made a relatively good recovery. Although he remains partially paralyzed, he can walk with a cane, and he retains his sense of humor and his interest in writing. But there was no way that his doctors could have known that. Like the Life Flight emergency rescue team, the emergency room team and neurosurgeons focused on saving his life and minimizing the secondary damage.

After the initial operation, the head-injured patient often needs more surgeries as the long, delicate, acute-care stage begins. Maintaining oxygen intake and controlling swelling continue to be key to survival and recovery, so the acute-care team hooks the patient to a respirator and administers diuretics to minimize fluid buildup. If this fails to control intracranial pressure, they may use barbiturates to put him or her into an artificial coma or give Pavulon (a long-acting muscle relaxant) combined with morphine as a sedative for inducing paralysis. Researchers aren't sure why these drugs sometimes work, but they suspect that slowing the body's functions reduces blood flow to the brain. The most recent treatment that shows promise in reducing swelling consists of lowering the brain's temperature by two degrees Fahrenheit.

Damage to the brain stem—the part of the brain that controls breathing, heart rate, blood pressure, and body temperature— means that the patient needs assistance with all these vital functions. Damage throughout the brain can disrupt the body's immune response, so fighting infection, from both penetrating wounds and surgery, is a major challenge. Traumatic brain injury patients often suffer epileptic seizures and a host of other medical complications that can demand months of acute care. After my childhood injury, I spent five weeks in the hospital. James Brady was in the hospital for eight months, Russell Moody, off and on for three years.

Often it is only after acute care is well under way that the medical team gets an inkling of the victim's chances for recovery. Some patients who early on look as though they'll do well slip into a coma and never regain consciousness. Others who are unresponsive suddenly and unexpectedly begin to improve. "You try not to get real hopeful with head injuries, because a lot of times, the results are pretty dismal," explains Dr. Harmann. "But when you do see someone respond to a verbal command the first time, everyone's elated."

EMTs, neurosurgeons, and emergency room doctors and nurses deal daily with head injury victims who look as though they will never regain what most of us agree is minimal human function— the ability to perceive and relate to what's going on around them, to feel love and pleasure, to communicate with others. In the cases of botched suicide attempts and octogenarians who have suffered serious falls, the temptation to be less aggressive in the battle for the patients' survival can be great. But absent written advance directives to the contrary, the team goes all out to save these lives.

A quarter of the victims of severe traumatic brain injury suffer lasting disabilities. In a 1984 report by the National Institute of Neurological Disorders and Stroke, only half of the survivors of serious head traumas had recovered well enough in three months' time to conduct the basic tasks of everyday life, such as feeding and bathing themselves, and to communicate with others. Of course, this doesn't suggest that they were back at their previous jobs or that they were entirely free of confusion, memory lapses, or emotional and sexual problems. Of the remainder, 35 percent experienced moderate disability: they were confined to a wheelchair, for example, or their speech was halting and slurred. Another 10 percent were severely disabled—conscious but completely dependent, with a serious loss in mental capacity. And 5 percent were in the ghostly limbo known as the persistent vegetative state.

Researchers are working on tests to predict a head injury patient's prognosis at various stages of treatment, but at this point all the available tests miss a substantial number who suddenly decline or improve. Of three patients rushed to the same hospital with apparently similar serious brain trauma, one may die of initial or secondary damage, another may be discharged conscious but severely disabled, and a third may recover well enough to live independently and hold a job. For the sake of that third patient, we don't want the trauma and acute-care professionals to give up—and even for the sake of that second patient. We can't judge what quality of life that survivor might find acceptable, and we can't know whether, given proper support and rehabilitation, he or she might continue to improve.

Most of the medical professionals who have worked with traumatic brain injuries have had all too many experiences like the one that Barbara Bowers had one night when she was flying with Life Flight. A group of teenagers in a pickup truck had been speeding along a narrow road through the beach resorts fifteen miles east of Galveston on the Bolivar Peninsula. None of them was wearing a seat belt. The driver lost control. In the horrific crash that followed, the kids were thrown out of the truck and onto the nearby fields and hedges. Bowers found one boy unconscious, inserted a nasal breathing tube, and got him back to the emergency room alive.

A few weeks later, while Bowers was sitting in her office, a colleague stuck her head in the door and announced that some people were there to see her. "It was the grandparents with this kid in a wheelchair," Bowers says. "All he could do was sit there and moan and cry. But the grandparents were so grateful that he was still alive. They came by because they wanted to thank me for saving him."

Although Bowers, who calls herself "a real quality-of-life person," found that experience upsetting, it didn't alter her determination to do everything she could to save the life of every injury victim that she was called upon to help. That was her mission. And, after all, she couldn't know what progress that kid might make in the coming weeks and months. A lot could depend on whether he had the insurance or other resources necessary to buy him the most appropriate, advanced rehabilitation.

Three decades ago, 90 percent of the victims of severe traumatic brain injury died. Now, thanks to the speed and sophistication of the treatment delivered from the accident scene through the acute-care phase, at least half live. As we shall see, responding to the needs of these survivors is a tremendous challenge that requires the concerted efforts of a great many people.

three

Hope on the Horizon

On the afternoon of June 4, 1996, an ambulance carried a coma-tose young piano teacher from Central Park, where she had been viciously beaten, to the emergency room of New York Hospital–Cornell Medical Center on New York City's Upper East Side. Her accused attacker, a mentally unbalanced and unemployed former sales clerk, had reportedly smashed her forehead on a concrete side-walk, shattering the bones above her right eye. He was said to have then turned her over and hammered her head against the pave-ment with such intensity that he fractured her skull behind her left ear. Although the neurosurgical resident on duty at the hospital in-serted a shunt to siphon off the excess fluid expected to build inside her skull from her battered and swelling brain, later that night her intracranial pressure rose precipitously anyway, threatening her life.

The physician in charge of the victim's case, Jam Ghajar, the chief of neurosurgery at Jamaica Hospital in Queens, ordered a CT scan, which showed an extensive clot building in her bruised right frontal cortex. Around midnight he drilled a small hole in her skull, and then, as he told Malcolm Gladwell (to whose thorough account of this case, in the July 8, 1996, *New Yorker,* I am indebted for the facts related here), "this big brain hemorrhage just came out—plop—like a big piece of black jelly." Five days later the patient developed a second clot, this time on the left temporal lobe, behind her left ear. This was an especially ominous development, since this area of the brain governs comprehension, and surgery to remove the clot might have inadvertently damaged the young woman's ability to speak and understand. Again an incision in her skull was made, and again, remarkably, the clot just plopped out on its own.

The young piano teacher has made remarkable progress but faces a long, arduous recovery and rehabilitation. But she was extremely lucky to have been taken to one of the few trauma centers in the country that specialize in traumatic brain injury. Five years earlier, when her chief physician and several other researchers had surveyed the nation's trauma centers, just one-third of them reported that they routinely monitored intracranial pressure. In other words, at most hospitals, the rising pressure inside her skull that twice led physicians to order CT scans, which discovered the blood clots and ultimately prompted life-saving surgery, might well have not been detected. Instead, she likely would have died.

In the years to come, many brain-injured victims across the country who formerly would have died may survive because they will receive treatment as good as that administered to the young piano teacher. If this happens, it will be in part because in the summer of 1993, following a professional meeting in Vancouver, Dr. Ghajar and two other neurosurgeons decided that something needed to be done to dramatically boost the grim odds facing comatose patients with traumatic brain injuries in the United States. About 40 percent of these people now die, while another 40 percent make a satisfactory recovery, which is usually defined as an outcome ranging from independent living with some disability to full recovery; the remaining 20 percent fall into a shadowy netherworld between persistent vegetative state and serious disability. The three physician-researchers enlisted the help of the Brain Trauma Foundation, the educational arm of the Aitken Neuroscience Institute, a research group of which Ghajar is president. (The institute was founded by the children of Prince Alfred von Auersperg and Sonny von Bulow, both of whom suffered fatal comas.)

The focus of the physicians' and the foundation's effort was to allow the thousands of U.S. hospitals that do not specialize in brain trauma to benefit from the experience of the handful of hospitals that do. At these few institutions, "it is now not unusual for the mortality rates of coma patients to run in the range of 20 percent or less," or half the deaths experienced at nonspecialist hospitals, Gladwell wrote in the *New Yorker*. Between winter 1994 and summer 1995, he continued, the foundation hosted eleven meetings featuring some of the world's leading specialists in brain injuries. At these grueling weekend sessions, the experts reviewed four thousand scientific papers relating to fourteen areas of brain-injury management.

The product of all this diligent work was a blue three-ring binder setting forth the scientific evidence and treatment guidelines for every phase of traumatic brain injury. Beginning in March 1996, the book was sent to every neurosurgeon in the United States; in addition, the Brain Trauma Foundation mailed it to scientific journals, hospitals, managed care groups, and insurance companies. This was, as Gladwell observed, the first organized effort by neurosurgeons to come up with a standardized set of state-of-the-art treatment recommendations for those with traumatic brain injuries. He estimated that if the guidelines "are adopted by anywhere close to a majority of the country's trauma centers, they could save more than 10,000 lives a year."

Though perhaps it could have happened a few years before it actually did, the fact that the nation's neurosurgeons only recently developed such a recommended treatment plan—or protocol, in medical jargon—is understandable. As Murray Goldstein, former director of the National Institute of Neurological Disorders and Stroke at the National Institutes of Health (NIH), noted just one year before the blue book was issued, "More has been learned in the past 20 years about how the human brain is organized and functions than in the past 200 years." He continued, "More has been learned in the past 10 years about nerve cell recovery from injury than in the past 10 centuries."

Now medical director for the United Cerebral Palsy Research and Educational Foundation, Goldstein elaborated on the progress in his foreword to the 1995 book *Brain Repair,* by Donald G. Stein, Simon Brailowsky, and Bruno Will: "Molecular genetics is describing the biological forces that determine the fundamental structures and functioning of the developing brain; behavioral neuroscience is describing the impact of the internal and external environments on the molding of behavior; and the clinical sciences are describing the impact of infection and injury to the brain on total body performance. Brain-imaging technologies are documenting how the living brain functions during the performance of the activities of daily living. The neurochemical processes controlling cognition including language, memory, and problem-solving are also being identified."

When Goldstein's former agency, the National Institute of Neurological Disorders and Stroke, was established in 1950, the conventional wisdom was that physicians would never be able to do much to help their brain-injured patients. Nerve cells, unlike skin and muscle tissue, were traditionally assumed to be incapable of repair or replication. Until recently, medical science held that once we reached adulthood, we had all the brain cells we would ever have and that any damaged or lost after that were gone forever. Congress, meanwhile, couldn't be persuaded to fund inquiries that seemed to have no potential for benefit.

But in the past few years, as Goldstein emphasizes, our understanding of the brain has undergone a revolution. New research findings promise hope for those suffering all sorts of neural damage, particularly for victims of brain trauma.

Neuroscientists have discovered that nerve cells, including brain cells, can regenerate when prompted by certain nerve growth factors. Indeed, traumatic brain injury itself appears to switch on genes that may trigger the release of these healing chemicals. One group of substances, gangliosides, which reside in the outer membranes of neurons, appear to cause the cells to sprout new branches that extend into neighboring areas of destruction and replace dead cells. Studies aimed at understanding and identifying such natural repair processes may enable doctors to help the brain reconstruct sections devastated by trauma. Research using fetal cell implants, which have shown promise in mending damaged spinal cords, may also have implications for traumatic brain injury. In either case, the information that had been contained in destroyed cells may have to be relearned, but some patients who now have limited potential for recovery might be able to eventually lead normal lives.

Both basic researchers, who unravel the mechanisms and study the chemicals by which the brain operates, and their clinical colleagues, who apply this knowledge to developing new therapies, have made breakthroughs that offer hope to present and future victims of severe brain trauma. For example, a blow to one part of the brain can trigger a massive release of normally well-controlled brain chemicals which, in turn, can damage sections of the brain not involved in the initial injury. Free radicals, amino acids, and perhaps even nitric oxide play a role in this secondary damage.

Once neuroscientists understand how and why this cascade of bio-chemical events occurs, clinical researchers may be able to develop drugs or other therapies to block this secondary physiological in-sult and prevent the cognitive and behavioral problems that it may cause down the line.

Another promising area of inquiry may one day limit the cel-lular devastation that brain injury leaves in its wake. For decades, physicians have used barbiturates to control the secondary dam-age that often follows the initial injury. But putting patients into a drug-induced coma carries its own risks. Moreover, doctors can't evaluate the recovery potential of a person in an artificial vegeta-tive state. Hypothermia—lowering the temperature of the brain—seems to provide similar benefits without some of the drawbacks. Researchers initially theorized that cooling slowed the metabolic rate, thus slowing brain activity. Now they believe that cooling sta-bilizes the blood vessels and inhibits the massive release of neuro-transmitters that set off a secondary chain of damaging events for brain-injured patients.

In 1995, the National Institutes of Health funded a $7.2 mil-lion, five-hundred-patient study to examine the benefits of hypo-thermia in those with severe traumatic brain injuries that result in coma. By late 1996, about two hundred of these patients had been treated and studied, including a post-treatment evaluation after six months. But because this is a completely blind experiment, no re-sults will be known until the study is complete in 1998. As I write, about three hundred additional patients are yet to be treated and examined at five medical centers nationwide. All patients in the study were to receive standardized, state-of-the-art treatment. But only half were to receive the experimental hypothermia treatment, thus permitting a statistical comparison of the efficacy of the inno-vative treatment versus that of the standard regimen.

According to the recipient of the NIH grant, Guy L. Clifton, hypothermia treatment should begin as soon as possible after injury and within six hours at the latest. Cooling blankets are wrapped around the patient to lower the body temperature to 90–91 degrees Fahrenheit (or 32–33 degrees Centigrade). This temperature is maintained for twenty-four hours. Then the patient is gradually warmed over twelve hours to normal body temperature.

The NIH grant came to Dr. Clifton, the chairman of neurosurgery at the UT-Houston Medical School of the University of Texas–Houston Health Science Center, because he and his colleagues had previously undertaken five years of preliminary clinical trials. These trials had been prompted by their earlier, encouraging laboratory studies indicating that decreasing the temperature within the skull by as little as two degrees may be effective in promoting recovery for those with brain trauma. The preliminary trials, which were run concurrently at Hermann Hospital in Houston and at Presbyterian Hospital in Pittsburgh, had suggested that use of hypothermia increased by 20 percent the number of patients achieving a good outcome—"good" being defined as a range of response, from being able to live independently with some residual disability to full recovery. That impressive numerical percentage, of course, represents an incalculable reduction in the toll of individual human suffering—by both patients and their families—not to mention significant savings in medical costs and in wages that would otherwise have been lost.

Another intriguing and seemingly promising approach to treating brain trauma involves hyperbaric therapy—administering high concentrations of oxygen under pressure. Medical science has long known that lack of oxygen is a major cause of secondary brain damage. Blot clots, for example, wreak only some of their havoc by compressing the tissue around them; they inflict far more harm by squeezing off blood vessels and thus depriving brain cells of oxygen. But just because too little oxygen harms brain cells, it doesn't necessarily follow that a large amount heals them. Yet that is precisely what the work done by clinical researcher Paul Harch of the Jo Ellen Smith Medical Center in New Orleans seems to indicate.

Dr. Harch has had some remarkable results treating brain-trauma patients with hyperbaric therapy. One instance involved a patient who had suffered a severe brain injury after jumping out of a car traveling forty-five miles per hour. A day after he was admitted to the hospital, the eighteen-year-old registered only seven out of a best possible score of fifteen on the Glasgow Coma Scale. Yet, ten weeks after hyperbaric treatment, he could walk on his own and talk. After one hundred treatments, the young man was transferred to a rehabilitation facility that didn't practice hyperbaric therapy; his progress plateaued. Four months later, he resumed hyperbaric therapy—and continued his recovery. Throughout the course of the case, Dr. Harch charted the healing of his patient's brain with SPECT scans, which use single photon emissions (SPEs) to create CT scan images. The scans showed that the area of injury had decreased in size. Within a year after his accident, the young man was running and riding a bicycle. Dr. Harch has found hyperbaric therapy effective even when it wasn't begun until months or even years after the trauma.

Although Dr. Harch has discussed his work at professional conferences, he has yet to publish a rigorous study with a broad enough patient population to give his work solid scientific underpinnings and thus to promote widespread use of hyperbaric therapy. Even the most impressive anecdotal successes are never enough to show a therapy to be effective, since so many factors—from physiological luck to the researcher's rapport with the patient—can come into play. But Dr. Harch's work may well indicate a hopeful new area of treatment, and other clinical scientists are waiting eagerly for the publication of his full study. Despite promising new research for treating acute brain injury, our ability to help survivors during rehabilitation hasn't kept pace with our skill at heroic rescue.

THE POLITICAL AWAKENING

Encouraging research discoveries, the general expansion of our knowledge about brain function, and good, old-fashioned political advocacy and lobbying to persuade legislators to deal decisively with the epidemic of brain trauma have finally begun to register in our national political consciousness. Unlike the Brain Trauma Foundation, which funded the brain-trauma protocol book and which sees its mission as mainly educational, the Brain Injury Association (BIA) has fought since its inception in 1980 to influence public policy on behalf of brain-trauma victims. To put itself where policy decisions are made, in 1990 this advocacy group moved its headquarters from Boston to Washington, D.C. In response to the BIA's efforts, in 1992 several U.S. senators and representatives introduced two bills aimed at dealing with traumatic brain injury— the first significant federal legislative action specifically targeted toward the epidemic. For two sessions, these bills worked their way through the tedious process of review and revision in each house of Congress. In 1996, one of them, the Traumatic Brain Injury Act, finally was approved by the Congress, was signed by President Clinton, and became law. It authorized the federal government to spend $24.5 million in the next three years on grants to states that developed model treatment programs as well as to federal agencies that studied the incidence of brain injuries and researched strategies for their prevention, treatment, and rehabilitation.

Thus far, the act has been more symbolic than substantive, since it authorized expenditures but didn't fund ongoing programs; funding must ultimately be fixed as a line item in a regular appropriation bill—something that has yet to happen. While much more public money is needed to fund research, the act is a welcome beginning.

Besides the Traumatic Brain Injury Act, a few other political steps in the right direction have been taken in the past few years. The Americans with Disabilities Act of 1990, for example, prohibits discrimination against people with many types of disabilities. By requiring that public buildings and public transportation be accessible to individuals in wheelchairs, this important law is making it easier for brain-injury victims with mobility problems to function independently.

THE REHABILITATION REVOLUTION

The Americans with Disabilities Act is especially important now, because in the area of traumatic brain injury, we are in the middle of a rehabilitation revolution. The great advances made in rehabilitative services are fortunate, since many people who formerly would have died of their brain injuries now survive thanks to advances in medicine and trauma care, and they therefore need help relearning skills and readjusting to life. The revolution began fairly quietly—indeed, it was virtually unnoticed by most citizens—in August 1950, when President Harry Truman established the predecessor of the National Institute of Neurological Disorders and Stroke. It slowly accelerated throughout the fifties, sixties, and seventies, despite the fact that treatments for diseases and disorders afflicting far fewer people than brain trauma does (such as muscular dystrophy and juvenile diabetes) received much more public attention and public money. And it began to pick up steam in 1989, when Congress and President George Bush declared the 1990s the Decade of the Brain—finally focusing national attention on unlocking the secrets of how the healthy brain develops and works and how the damaged brain might be restored.

Since 1980 therapeutic techniques have advanced dramatically, and the number of brain-injury inpatient rehabilitation facilities has increased more than a hundredfold. In the past ten years alone, according to the National Conference of State Legislatures (NCSL), the for-profit brain-injury rehabilitation industry has grown exponentially to the point where it now generates an estimated $10 billion in fees annually. Still, the NCSL calculates that only one in twenty people with brain injuries receives the rehabilitation services that he or she needs.

What typically stands in a patient's way is not the lack of appropriate programs but the patient's inability to pay for them. For those who are not insured, have exhausted their insurance benefits, or have left rehabilitation facilities to live with their families or in the community, state services are often grossly inadequate, terribly fragmented, and shamefully inefficient. A number of state bureaucracies have no central headquarters to which people with traumatic brain injuries can turn. State services are spread throughout myriad agencies and departments, from health and education departments to mental health and social services. This forces the already highly stressed victims of brain injury—or, more likely, members of their equally stressed families—to go, hat in hand, from office to office in a frustrating and frequently fruitless effort to find the services that they need. This fragmentation also has a debilitating effect on the states themselves by handicapping their policy makers' efforts to gather the data necessary to develop programs, procedures, and systems that would better meet the needs of victims of brain trauma.

Yet in recent years a few bright spots have begun to emerge. Many states are attempting to improve how they serve people with brain injuries by establishing state councils, creating lead agencies, and instituting a system called case management to control costs by ensuring that people get the most appropriate services. These services are paid for through traditional sources of financing, such as Medicaid, vocational rehabilitation grants, and state general-revenue funds, and sometimes through more innovative financing approaches. Some states, for example, have established dedicated reserves funded by fines for such motor vehicle violations as speeding, drunk driving, or failure to use safety belts.

A couple of progressive states have taken the lead in setting up comprehensive model programs that others already have begun to emulate. The case management system mentioned above, for instance, was developed in Minnesota and is employed effectively in Florida as well. It holds particular promise because it recognizes that each brain trauma and each brain-trauma victim are different and that both the potential level of recovery and the time required to reach it vary from person to person.

Under a case management system, families that are able and willing still provide their brain-injured members with such necessities as food and shelter, but they receive help that lets them do so without necessarily sacrificing some of their members' lives to full-time caring for the victim. For example, day care for the brain injured can enable a mother, father, or spouse to continue working. And with a job-training program combined with a transportation service, even a moderately disabled brain-injured person may eventually be able to contribute to his or her living expenses.

Case managers are trained to match brain-injured individuals and their families with the services that they need and to make those services accessible to them. Case management not only assures more appropriate treatment; it also costs less than the traditional—and haphazard—methods of distributing aid. Thus, by focusing on home- and community-based programs rather than residential treatment institutions, Minnesota estimates that it saves $1 million a year.

But as important as life-saving treatment and rehabilitation are for dealing with brain trauma, one thing is even more crucial: prevention. There, too, our first small steps already have begun to make a difference. The lion's share of the 2 million Americans who suffer traumatic brain injuries each year sustain them in automobile wrecks. Not only do seat belts and shoulder harnesses save lives; they also have significantly reduced the number of accident victims who suffer brain traumas. Unfortunately, however, only the District of Columbia and eleven states allow police officers to stop vehicles solely for seat-belt violations: California, Connecticut, Georgia, Hawaii, Iowa, Louisiana, New Mexico, New York, North Carolina, Oregon, and Texas. Tougher laws and stepped-up enforcement would certainly boost compliance in the other four states—and lead to an accompanying reduction in brain injuries and deaths.

Air bags, which are now standard equipment in most new cars and which federal safety standards require to be installed in all new passengers cars and light trucks by 1999, are estimated to have saved nine hundred lives from the late 1980s to 1994, according to the National Center for Statistics and Analysis of the National Highway Traffic Safety Administration. Air bags have also greatly reduced traumatic brain injuries among front-seat passengers involved in head-on crashes and, in the case of vehicles that have side-mounted air bags, among those hit from the side as well.

In late 1995, a troubling trend emerged. In November, the U.S. Centers for Disease Control and Prevention (CDC) noted in the *Morbidity and Mortality Weekly Report* that eight infants and children, front-seat passengers all, had sustained traumatic brain and other injuries as a result of the impact from suddenly inflating air bags. By 1997 a national controversy had developed, and it can only be described as curious: whereas air bags could be blamed for sixty-one fatalities (most of them preventable), air bags had saved more than sixteen hundred lives. Air bags have clearly been of significant value in protecting adult and teenage car passengers. But after discovering that some parents were not heeding the warnings printed on many child safety seats and on places like the visors of cars equipped with air bags, the CDC, quite appropriately, underscored several important recommendations for children:

- All infants and children should be properly restrained in child safety seats or with lap and shoulder belts.
- All infants and children should ride only in the back seats of cars, and infants under twenty pounds or one year of age should ride in rear-facing safety seats mounted in the back seats only. The last point is especially important: infants in rear-facing safety seats should never be placed in the front seats of cars or trucks with passenger-side air bags.
- If a car does not have a rear seat, a child riding in the front seat should be positioned as far away from the air bag as possible.

By late 1997 the air bag controversy remained unresolved. Opponents have gained the right to disconnect air bags that might harm small or frail persons; proponents lobby for both front- and side-mounted air bags. At the moment, there is one new and promising passive safety feature that may reduce the number of two-car accidents: daytime running lights. The straightforward reasoning for this innovation is that using headlights makes cars more conspicuous during daylight hours, making others—drivers and pedestrians alike—more aware of approaching vehicles. Many manufacturers are beginning to make running lights that are activated by ignition switches standard equipment on their vehicles. If one doesn't own a new car with this feature, the same safety advantage can be achieved simply by turning the lights on manually (although of course one must then remember to turn them off while turning off the ignition in order to avoid risking a dead battery). For now, taking advantage of this commonsense expedient seems reasonable—as does anything else that improves one's odds of avoiding a traffic accident, from slowing down on wet roads to leaving ten minutes earlier than necessary to reach your destination. Whether use of daytime running lights actually will pan out as projected—particularly whether the strategy will remain successful when all cars on the road during the day have their headlights on and people have become accustomed to that sight—is something that only time and further research will tell us.

Another life- and brain-saving expedient about which there is little scientific debate involves those who ride on motorcycles. A proven, highly effective way of reducing crash-related head injuries—the main cause of death among unhelmeted motorcyclists—is requiring all motorcycle drivers and passengers of whatever age to wear helmets. Helmets are 67 percent effective at preventing brain injuries, the National Highway Safety Administration estimates, and where they are required by law, the number of motorcyclists using them approaches 100 percent.

The good news is that as of July 1, 1997, twenty-five states and the District of Columbia had motorcycle helmet laws that applied to all riders, while twenty-two other states had such laws affecting only some riders, usually those under eighteen; Colorado, Illinois, and Iowa had no helmet laws at all. But there is bad news on this subject as well. This is an instance of our nation taking one step forward after we took two steps back, and as I write we are starting to go backward once again. To understand how and why, we need to be aware of a little history.

Before 1967, only three states had motorcycle helmet laws. That year the federal government began requiring states to enact such laws in order to qualify for certain highway construction funds and federal safety program grants. By 1975, all but three states had laws requiring motorcyclists of all ages to wear helmets. Then, starting in 1976, the federal Department of Transportation (DOT) began to financially penalize states without so-called universal helmet laws. State governments promptly began to pressure Congress to revoke the DOT's authority to assess penalties for noncompliance.

Congress caved in to the pressure, with predictable results. Once the federal sanctions were gone, motorcyclists continued to intensely lobby state legislators to eliminate or soften the helmet laws, often organizing politically and pressing for antihelmet resolutions at precinct, county, and state Republican and Democratic party conventions. As a consequence, between 1976 and 1978, nineteen states weakened their helmet laws, applying them only to young riders, typically those under age eighteen.

Why did so many motorcyclists oppose being forced to protect their heads? Perhaps the answer is the simple truth that motorcyclists are a notoriously independent breed, more adventuresome and tolerant of risk than most of the rest of us, and many of them tend to see helmets as both a symbolic and concrete example of a bothersome government interfering with their freedom to let the wind blow through their hair—one of the great sensual pleasures, along with the intense physical "rush" of speed generally, that goes with motorcycle riding. After all, motorcyclists face a risk of death and injury that is twenty times higher per mile traveled than that experienced by people in cars. (This is a statistic that the government should require be part of all published and broadcast advertising for motorcycles, much like the surgeon general's health warnings are printed on cigarette packages.)

All this is not to say that motorcyclists have not presented some superficially plausible safety arguments against helmets over the years. Some motorcyclists, for instance, have claimed that helmets restrict their hearing and peripheral vision. A 1995 study shows that full-coverage helmets do indeed curtail one's horizontal peripheral vision, but only to a minor degree—about 3 percent. Riders easily compensated for that, the study found, by rotating their heads more to look around before changing lanes. The same study found no restriction in the helmeted riders' ability to hear horn signals or see vehicles in adjacent lanes before changing lanes. Additionally, some motorcyclists critical of helmet laws have cited a study showing that helmets cause neck injuries, possibly by adding to the head mass in a crash. But a dozen other studies refute that finding.

When motorcyclists' deaths and injuries began to climb after their success in weakening helmet laws, a more rational view started to prevail in some places. Between 1980 and the early 1990s, several of the states that had previously watered down their laws reinstated helmet laws for all riders. In 1991, meanwhile, Congress enacted the bureaucratically titled Intermodal Surface Transportation Efficiency Act, which established incentives for states to approve seatbelt and helmet laws covering everyone. Those states that had enacted both such laws were eligible for special federal safety grants, but those that didn't have both laws on their books by October 1993 had up to 3 percent of their federal highway funds diverted to highway safety programs.

Then in the anti-Washington, antiregulatory fervor after the Republicans seized control of both the House and the Senate in 1994, Congress once again flip-flopped. In the fall of 1995, the national legislature lifted the sanctions against states without laws that required motorcyclists to wear helmets. This opened the door for states to once again repeal universal helmet laws. Congress's zigging and zagging underscores how hard it sometimes is for us as a society to apply the measures that many of us already know will work to prevent traumatic brain injury. And it illustrates why everyone who cares about this issue needs to get involved politically—from writing letters to legislators and local newspapers to joining with advocacy groups like the Brain Injury Association.

The plain fact is, preventive measures like helmet laws are useful in reducing deaths and traumatic brain injuries. Take the experience in Texas, where I now live. From 1968 to 1977, Texas law mandated that every motorcyclist and passenger wear a helmet. That law is estimated to have saved 650 lives—and who knows how many brains from being battered. But in 1977 the law was softened and made to apply only to riders younger than eighteen. The weakened statute coincided with a 35 percent rise in motorcyclist deaths. Nonetheless, the news of this increase did not get adequately communicated, nor did the rise in carnage and scrambled brains change peoples' behavior. By August 1989, only 41 percent of Texas's motorcyclists were said to be using helmets. When Texas reinstated its universal helmet law in September 1989, the numbers of helmet wearers rose to 90 percent in the first month that the law was in effect. The compliance rate was 98 percent by June 1990. Meanwhile, serious-injury crashes per registered motorcycle dropped by 11 percent. Similar positive results were seen in other states that have likewise reinstituted laws requiring helmets on all motorcycle riders. By 1997 Texas lawmakers decided that only riders under twenty-one would be required to wear helmets. Fatalities and injuries will inevitably increase, as will the public cost of motorcycle crashes.

The nation also has begun, ever so slowly, to recognize that bicycle helmets also prevent brain and other injuries and thus that bike riders should wear helmets, too. In 1995, the Centers for Disease Control and Prevention reported that each year, nearly 1,000 Americans die from injuries caused by bicycle crashes and 550,000 are treated annually in emergency rooms for bike-related injuries. It observed that head injuries account for 62 percent of the bicycle-related deaths and for 33 percent of the bike-related emergency room visits. And it noted that 7 percent of all brain injuries result from bike accidents. Moreover, the CDC cited a 1991 study from the *Journal of the American Medical Association,* which concluded that universal use of bicycle helmets in the United States could spare us an average of 500 fatal and 151,400 nonfatal head injuries every year. Based on these findings and others — including a case-controlled study in Seattle that found helmet use can cut the risk of bicycle-related head injury by 74 to 85 percent — the CDC recommended that helmets be worn by bicyclists of all ages and at all times whenever they ride. It also urged states and communities to enact laws and implement education campaigns designed to encourage helmet use.

Between July 1991 and March 1997, twelve communities placed on the books comprehensive ordinances requiring all riders to wear helmets. Beginning in 1990, sixteen other jurisdictions passed laws requiring helmets on bike riders under sixteen or eighteen. As of 1997, however, no state had a universal helmet law for bicyclists. But fifteen states have enacted half-a-loaf bike helmet laws, the first of which took effect in July 1992. This patchwork of legislation includes statutes requiring helmets on people below the ages of eighteen (California), seventeen (Florida), sixteen (Alabama, Delaware, Georgia, Maryland, and Oregon), fifteen (West Virginia), fourteen (New Jersey and New York), thirteen (Massachusetts), twelve (Connecticut and Pennsylvania), and eight (Rhode Island). At least these laws do affect the largest group of people who ride bicycles — children and teenagers. And thus they represent a hopeful beginning — but only a beginning (and usually a lightly enforced one at that) — toward what should be mandatory helmet use by everyone who climbs onto a bicycle.

Prevention is not limited to drivers and passengers of cars, bikes, and motorcycles. Other innovative efforts include a model program by Seattle's Harborview Injury Prevention and Research Center (HIPRC) — a collaboration between the Harborview Medical Center and the University of Washington Medical School and School of Public Health and Community Medicine — to encourage horseback riders to wear helmets. HIPRC helped to design an improved equestrian helmet that costs only half the price of earlier models; it also aided in a promotion supplying discount coupons for the helmets. And it assisted in forming a national coalition of more than a dozen organizations—among them the American Academy of Pediatrics, the U.S. Combined Training Association, 4-H, the U.S. Pony Club, and the national SAFE KIDS campaigns—to encourage use of equestrian helmets.

Indeed, among the most hopeful events of the past decade or so is the creation of injury prevention and research centers like the one in Seattle; there are seven others nationwide. These organizations research the causes and effects of injuries and then attempt to apply what they learn toward developing community programs that can stop injuries before they happen.

Take, for instance, the all-too-frequent tragedy of kids being hit by cars, a dispiriting staple of local television's evening news broadcasts. In most U.S. cities and in the country as a whole, such car-pedestrian accidents kill more children from ages five to fourteen than do any other type of accident, and they leave many other kids living with the often-debilitating consequences of traumatic brain injury. But it is no longer the top cause of death for such youngsters in Seattle. The reason is the enlightened efforts of HIPRC's Prevention and Health Promotion Section, where researchers develop and evaluate injury-prevention strategies, institute programs, and also spread the word about how often certain injuries occur and how much they cost, both economically and in human suffering.

To grapple with the problem of children being hit by cars, the researchers first studied a number of Seattle's previous fatal car-pedestrian accidents involving children. The aim was to find out exactly who was most at risk and why. The researchers discovered that frequently drivers couldn't see the children or had an obstructed view prior to hitting them. And they also learned that about half the preschooler pedestrians killed by cars were struck at home—in the garage or driveway. Moreover, when the researchers interviewed parents, they found that the parents usually thought that their kids were much more streetwise about cars and traffic than the researchers determined the children actually were.

Armed with this evidence, the researchers designed a comprehensive child-pedestrian safety program. The cornerstone of this venture is an instructional plan used to teach street safety to kids in elementary schools, one which involves parents in the project. The program works. Research shows that it does improve children's ability to cross streets safely.

The HIPRC researchers also found that children living in apartment complexes, housing projects, and similar multifamily dwellings were nearly six times more likely to be hit by a car than were kids living in single-family residences. Such multifamily complexes, they discovered, often lack sufficient playground space and also tend to be located in areas with busier streets, higher speed limits, and denser on-street parking.

Working with the Seattle police and the city engineering department, the researchers recommended traffic safety measures aimed at improving pedestrian safety at crosswalks, where 30 percent of the pedestrian accidents in Seattle occur. The engineers put up new warning signs. The police strictly enforced laws requiring drivers to stop when pedestrians were in crosswalks and issued a record number of forty-seven-dollar traffic tickets when drivers didn't stop. Yet the four-year project demonstrated that the hardest thing to change is drivers' reckless behavior. By the end of the study, many drivers were still whizzing through crosswalks while children were in them.

Despite that hitch, which shows the need for more innovative strategies or stiffer fines and tougher policing or both, there is no doubt that, overall, Seattle's program for teaching kids to be safer pedestrians saves children's lives and prevents many traumatic brain injuries. For that reason, the program—which is available on computer disc from HIPRC—is endorsed by the National Highway Traffic Safety Administration and the federal Bureau of Maternal and Child Health. But the program is also an admirable, working example epitomizing the central mission and message of all eight injury prevention centers around the country, which together are working to explode the myth—and it is a myth—that nothing can be done to prevent accidents. "Simply put," as the Seattle center tells a public that is still all too indifferent, "the primary cause of accidents is our fatalistic acceptance of them."

The Rough Road to Rehabilitation

Given prompt and appropriate trauma and acute care, a small percentage of victims of serious traumatic brain injury (no one is sure quite how many) recover virtually all their faculties on their own. Some cases of recovery are so remarkable that they border on the bizarre. During a June 1993 arrow-throwing tournament near Montana's Little Bighorn River, a five-foot-long arrow lodged in the head of a Crow boy who was playing nearby. (Crow arrows are thrown by hand rather than shot from a bow.) Three days later, doctors said that the nine-year-old's only lasting disability might be partial loss of sight.

From the beginning, luck plays a huge part in healing the damage caused by traumatic brain injuries. Like the man who shot the nail into his brain (Chapter 1), the Crow boy was physiologically lucky. Because the missiles causing their head injuries broke through their skulls, pressure didn't build to the point where it cut off blood flow, yet they escaped the major secondary risk in penetrating wounds—infection. And either the missiles that injured them didn't damage crucial areas or the brain was able to repair itself or reroute functions, as it sometimes does, to cells that had escaped unscathed.

Other victims of head trauma benefit from a different kind of luck: their accidents occur in the right place at the right time.

At the height of the Hollywood Harley-Davidson fad of the late 1980s, actor Gary Busey was an enthusiastic motorcyclist who loved feeling the wind in his hair. In fact, the Oscar-nominated star of *The Buddy Holly Story* raised money to lobby successfully against California's mandatory helmet bill. When he lost control of his Harley around noon on a Sunday in 1988, he wasn't wearing a helmet. The back of his head smashed into a curb. After ninety minutes of surgery to remove blood clots, he was placed on the critical list in the intensive care unit; yet a week later, a spokesman for Cedars-Sinai Medical Center pronounced him "out of the woods." Busey recovered completely, but he did change his position regarding protective headgear. "Next time you're doing forty-five miles per hour, look at the curb and think about slam-dancing with it once, and you'll start thinking about helmets," he told viewers of the *Arsenio Hall Show*.

Busey was lucky. His traumatic brain injury occurred in the middle of the day with plenty of people around to summon emergency medical technicians, who stabilized him and rushed him to one of the world's most advanced neurotrauma centers, which happened to be nearby. Had he dropped his cycle on a remote mountain road or late at night on a quiet suburban street, he might well have suffered irreversible brain damage.

Stories of the less lucky seldom make a news splash unless, like the Nancy Cruzan case, they create precedent-setting legal conflicts. Yet every month or so, a national magazine, wire service, or local television station will carry a story about someone who "miraculously" recovers from severe head trauma. Such accounts make perennially good copy.

Why do we celebrate the lucky ones, those who beat the overwhelming odds against them? Part of the reason is that is the definition of news: the rare, the unusual, the unexpected. But I think there is another reason as well: everybody loves a lottery. Despite the staggering odds against winning, millions of us buy tickets. Because someone usually does win, I can hope that the next winner will be me. Matters of luck generate hope, and hope produces optimism. I think we like to be reminded that, just as we are all vulnerable to misfortunes, accidents and injuries among them, unpredictable good fortune may strike us as well. By combining both the bad luck and the good in one tale, stories of quick and total recovery from life-threatening trauma reassure us that we can be lucky, too.

Unfortunately, years of reading uplifting articles about miraculous recoveries may lead us to think of traumatic brain injury as less devastating than it often is. Media coverage of medical advances primes us to expect that doctors and hospitals can quickly and accurately diagnose any anomaly and fix any abnormality. We must acknowledge the importance of individual cases of recovery, but we mustn't lose sight of the profound problems that afflict less fortunate victims and the enormous challenge that traumatic brain injury presents to our entire society.

Another problem with these stories is that they often gloss over the hard work that combines with luck to produce those "miracles." On June 6, 1994, the front page of the metro section of the *Houston Chronicle* carried a feature headlined "Miracle at Scarborough High." It reported the graduation with honors of Julie Cervantes, who had spent three months in a persistent vegetative state following a car accident during her junior year. Only a small quadrant of a wheelchair wheel is visible in the photograph of the proud graduate in her cap and gown, who triumphantly holds her diploma aloft. The story waits almost to the end to tell us that Cervantes was never able to return to classes on campus (she completed her junior and senior years through the Houston Independent School District's homebound program) and that her need for speech and physical therapy is a continuing one. A casual reading leaves the impression that after barely two years of determined effort, family and community support, and faith, she now leads a normal life. But although she has accomplished a lot against great odds, Julie Cervantes still has a long, rough road ahead.

According to the Brain Injury Association, the average victim of severe brain trauma who is fortunate enough to survive and regain consciousness faces five to ten years of demanding, expensive, often frustrating rehabilitation. Even that investment carries no guarantee of ultimately achieving independence, much less complete recovery.

One distinguishing tenet of American culture is the conviction that anyone can beat the odds simply by trying hard enough and having the right attitude. Some of us like to say that people create their own luck. But when we utter that aphorism, we may be confusing luck with achievement. Luck just happens, by chance or fortuity; achievement is the result of talent, effort, commitment—and the ability to recognize and seize the opportunities that luck brings our way. We may also want to believe that we create our own luck because we yearn for control. To the extent that we think we can manipulate luck, we feel less vulnerable to outside forces, more capable of controlling our own destinies.

We admire and sometimes designate as heroes individuals who are upbeat despite adversity, who retain humor and determination in the face of such terrible luck as a severe traumatic brain injury. Their ability to smile and joke helps us to get beyond, even to deny, their severe handicaps. We can forget how hard they struggle to achieve simple things that we take for granted. Although we know that they suffer, we can turn our attention away from their distress, denying or ignoring their loss of capacity, function, and opportunity. Or we can transform their plight into a source of inspiration. An individual bearing serious disability with such grace makes our own lesser adversities seem insignificant.

In one sense, former White House press secretary James Brady was profoundly unlucky in March 1981; he caught a bullet intended for his boss, President Ronald Reagan. In another respect, Brady was lucky, because he was surrounded by Secret Service agents trained in crisis response. He reached the emergency room within ten minutes of being shot. He was conscious until he was anesthetized, less than an hour after he was shot, for surgery to remove blood clots and most of the four or five large fragments of the "devastator" bullet that John Hinckley had fired into his brain.

Although his neurosurgeon gave him only a one-in-ten chance of surviving the injury, Brady pulled through. A few hours after surgery, he obeyed a command to squeeze his wife's hand. The following day, he tossed a ball around the intensive care unit. Within three days, he was telling jokes; within ten, he was phoning his office. Brady retained his detailed memory for past events and his keen interest in the news, and he was able to begin physical, speech, and occupational therapy a week after his injury. His medical recovery was remarkable.

But severed arteries in the left hemisphere, combined with the damage that the bullet inflicted directly on the left frontal lobe and on the right parietal lobe, just under the crown of his skull, left Brady with permanent brain damage. Even given all his good luck, the determined and effective support of his wife, Sarah, the resources that powerful connections made available, and his own optimism and sense of humor, Brady suffered lasting disabilities from his traumatic brain injury. Despite six years of intensive rehabilitation, he remained partially paralyzed on his left side. Ten years after the shooting, he could walk 150 yards a day with a leg brace and cane. He still had difficulty with short-term memory and with judging time.

For the first two years, Brady had assumed that if he worked hard enough at his rehabilitation, he eventually would recover all his functions. When he realized in the summer of 1983 that he would never get much better than he was then, he sank into a deep depression. Retaining his title as White House press secretary and returning to work for a few hours a week the next fall helped him to emerge, but he became bored with the small tasks assigned to him. Thousands of people he didn't know sent Brady get-well cards, but many of his friends and colleagues avoided him, unable to cope with his physical disabilities and his shaky voice, not to mention the emotional unsteadiness that is a frequent side effect of the kind of brain damage that Brady suffered. After years of turning down offers of positions with various organizations for the disabled, Brady agreed to become the spokesperson for the Brain Injury Association.

The Brain Injury Association (BIA) is a group founded by Massachusetts real estate broker Marilyn Spivack as the National Head Injury Foundation in 1980, when she was unable to find a suitable rehabilitation program for her brain-injured twenty-one-year-old daughter. At the time, the United States had only seven facilities specializing in helping victims of brain trauma recover function. The BIA predicts that by 1998 there will be more than one thousand. Part of the credit for this increase belongs to BIA, which has brought national awareness to this previously silent epidemic. As I have noted, the BIA has helped to persuade state and federal lawmakers to pass legislation aimed at preventing brain trauma, to designate funds for promising research, to increase services for the brain-injured, and to see that the people who can best benefit from these services receive them (Chapter 3).

Even for victims of traumatic brain injury who have access to appropriate services, the five- or ten-year road through intensive rehabilitation is long, uphill, winding, and cluttered with obstacles. The way is always rough and sometimes impassable. In any individual case, no one knows how far it will extend before it ends in a sheer wall or even a drop-off. Each year, traumatic brain injury leaves between seventy thousand and ninety thousand Americans with serious disabilities. Even with excellent rehabilitative treatment, they still may never be able to walk across a room, follow the plot of a simple television program, speak at normal speed, or recognize that they should put on a sweater or jacket before venturing out in thirty-degree weather.

When someone who was expected to die not only survives but recovers enough to live independently, we can all feel that the enormous investment of time, resources, and effort was worth it. But often before the patient reaches that goal, recovery slows and stops—or even goes backward. For example, a stroke or a seizure can cause dramatic deterioration in someone who has been making progress. Nancy Cruzan's doctors thought she was improving until some medical or neurological event—no one is sure just what—sent her into a permanent vegetative state. Recovery doesn't follow a single or simple pattern, and that uncertainty adds to the burden that traumatic brain injury places on everyone it touches.

Following the 1985 car accident that left him severely brain-damaged, nineteen-year-old Brian Rife spent 180 days in a vegetative state. When he finally regained consciousness, his first words —halting, so far from normal speech as to sound like almost meaningless vocalizations—were "I go home."

But Brian was nowhere near well enough to go home. He faced a long struggle to regain his sense of the world and his ability to communicate his own thoughts and feelings. And his family faced a struggle of their own: to keep him in Virginia's Mount Vernon

Hospital, where he could get the rehabilitation services that he needed and still be close enough for them to visit regularly. Brian had developed bonds with the therapists on Mount Vernon's staff; he trusted and felt comfortable with them. Sending him to another facility would fracture the fragile contacts that gave him essential support in the tough, repetitious tasks that made up his tedious, exhausting daily climb out of the abyss of isolation and confusion. Yet Mount Vernon's program cost eighteen thousand dollars per month, and the Rifes' insurance was running out. Medicaid would take over, but Medicaid wanted to send him to another facility. Finally, through a letter-writing campaign to state officials, his mother, Janet, won the battle to keep Brian in place.

Janet Rife's victory only bought her son the help he needed to travel as far as he was able along the rough road to recovery. It didn't guarantee how far he would go. It was ten months after the accident before doctors removed the tracheotomy tube that had helped him breathe without choking on his own saliva. A week later, he began eating soft food. At eleven months, he was just beginning to learn how to operate a wheelchair. His doctors were sure that his hearing and vision were permanently impaired, but now that he had emerged from a vegetative state, they couldn't predict how much further he was capable of going. They warned his family that the chances of his being able to hold a job, take care of all his daily needs, or walk were remote.

"At this point, I'm very accepting of Brian as he is," Janet Rife told a friend in 1986. "You make peace with what you've got. When I hug him and kiss him, it sure is better than visiting his grave." Eleven years later, Brian still struggles to regain lost capacities.

Although the road to recovery varies from patient to patient, the milestones look similar along the way. Most victims who arrive at the hospital unconscious but who ultimately improve pass through the eight stages delineated by the Rancho Los Amigos Cognitive

Scale. (The scale shown here was prepared by the Professional Staff Association, Rancho Los Amigos Hospital, Downey, California.) Many of these patients stall or stop along the way. The straightforward descriptions of the challenges and torments faced by patients at each level read like a painful psychological climb out of Dante's Inferno—only internal and in reverse.

Rancho Los Amigos Cognitive Scale
1. No response: unresponsive to any stimulus.
2. Generalized response: limited, inconsistent, nonpurposeful responses, often to pain only.
3. Localized response: purposeful responses; may follow simple commands; may focus on presented object.
4. Confused, agitated: heightened state of activity; confused, disoriented; aggressive behavior; unable to perform self-care; unaware of present events; agitation appears related to internal confusion.
5. Confused, inappropriate: nonagitated; appears alert; responds to commands; distractible; does not concentrate on tasks; agitated responses to external stimuli; verbally inappropriate; does not learn new information.
6. Confused, appropriate: good directed behavior, needs cueing; able to relearn old skills as activities of daily living (ADLs); serious memory problems; some awareness of self and others.
7. Automatic, appropriate: appears appropriately oriented; frequently robotlike in daily routine; minimal or absent confusion; shallow recall; increased awareness of self, interaction in environment; lacks insight into condition; decreased judgment and problem solving; unable to plan realistically for future.
8. Purposeful, appropriate: alert, oriented; recalls and integrates past events; learns new activities and can continue without supervision; independent in home and living skills; capable of driving; defects in stress tolerance, judgment, abstract reasoning persist; may function at reduced levels in society.

Russell Moody lingered for a month at level 1, for another at level 2. After another six weeks, he reached level 3. Then he slipped back and became unresponsive to commands. For six months in all, he hovered at or near a vegetative state.

"It was an earthshaking thing for me to make a decision, was Russell better off dead or alive?" his father, Bobby Moody, told an interviewer for the PBS documentary *Broken Rhymes*. Released in 1983, three years after Moody's near-fatal auto accident, the film follows his early rehabilitation and the rehabilitations of three other young, male brain-trauma victims: Mark Barton, a promising high school athlete injured in a fall; Carlos Risker, a young electronics designer struck by a bus; and David Rizek, a brilliant law student left brain-damaged by a mugger. The other three were all further along in their recoveries than Moody. They were relearning the skills of everyday living, dealing with their emotional reactions in group therapy sessions, and actively struggling to reestablish themselves as adults. "It's like switching from automatic transmission down to a manual," Risker explained, describing his problems mastering ordinary, routine tasks like using a washing machine.

Five years after his injury, Barton was volunteering part-time at a Montessori school, rather than attending college as he had hoped to do. He seemed to have a special rapport with the children, helping them learn for the first time the basic cognitive skills, like shape identification, that he himself had relearned so recently. "The word 'rehabilitation' is like a dream, because it means getting back like you were," he said. "You can't ever get back like you were. 'Rehabilitation' in my sense means making something of your life."

Although the complexity of the law and the verbal quickness needed to be a lawyer were beyond Rizek, he was able to handle a job doing searches for a title company. His mother told the interviewer that she yearned for the day when he would be able to live on his own. Her plight reflected that of other parents of brain-trauma victims who had just reached the brink of adulthood when a head injury knocked them back to childlike dependency.

At the time of the film, these three young men were miles farther along the rehabilitation path than Moody. In one scene shot through a two-way mirror, he stared into the camera with haunted eyes, his head and upper body listing to the left. The narrator, actor Richard Burton, muses, "Is Russell Moody in there, looking for a way back to where we are?"

That way led through the rehabilitation program at Houston's Medical Center del Oro, where Moody intermittently spent three years. His progress was interrupted by periodic transfers back to John Sealy Hospital at the University of Texas Medical Branch in Galveston to deal with the continuing medical problems that complicated his course of recovery. Fortunately, apart from his brain injury, he hadn't suffered other serious damage; many other people whose head traumas come from vehicular accidents aren't so lucky.

For the first week after his injury, doctors had kept Moody in a barbiturate coma to control the potentially lethal pressure inside his skull. Neuroscientists don't know exactly how barbiturates do this, but they theorize that keeping the brain as inactive as possible reduces swelling. For the next four months, Moody remained at or below seven on the Glasgow Coma Scale. He suffered fevers and ear infections. Once he began responding, Moody had to learn to swallow—first consciously, then automatically—before he could learn to make the voluntary sounds that, with great effort, he would develop into comprehensible speech. He had to relearn to grasp things with his hands and to sit up.

Angry outbursts are typical of the severely brain-injured, and Moody displayed those—but, remarkably, he also maintained his sense of humor. In the film, which was shot two years into his journey through rehabilitation, one of his nurses asked him if he remembered how he used to bite her fingers when she used a tongue depressor to examine his mouth. "That was the only thing that gave me pleasure," he responded, incredibly slowly, sounding like an old 45-rpm record playing at 33 rpm. "The only thing was, I should have seasoned your fingers."

The documentary made poignantly clear how much easier it would have been for Moody to allow himself to slip back into a more muffled awareness, a passive relationship with his surroundings, rather than keep struggling to advance, inch by inch, toward independence. One of the greatest rehabilitation hurdles is exhaustion. For victims of traumatic brain injury, consciousness, let alone the focus and concentration that learning requires, demands a huge effort. Three or four hours a day is the most that they can manage.

Five years after Moody's car wreck, his MRI showed extensive loss of brain tissue in his right parietal and temporal lobes. He could walk with two canes and a leg brace and could get himself into and out of his wheelchair. His speech was intelligible but slow; he scored only in the fifth percentile for young adults in word retrieval. His recognition of drawings of plants and animals was slightly impaired. He suffered from migraines, and he was on anticonvulsants to control the epilepsy that plagued him, as it does many head trauma victims. He hadn't shown much cognitive improvement in a year. In the opinion of the team treating him at Medical Center del Oro, Moody had reached a rehabilitation plateau.

From the moment that Russell was rushed from the scene of his Jeep accident to the trauma center, his father had been determined to give him every possible chance at recovery. Bobby Moody had the means to pay for the best care available, and his strong Methodist faith backed his determination with optimism, pragmatism, and spiritual support. He found appropriate rehabilitation services located only an hour away in Houston, but he couldn't locate anyplace in the region to offer Russell what he would need next—training in the skills of independent living. So the Moody Foundation, the family's philanthropic arm, established the Transitional Learning Center (TLC) in Galveston to help Russell and others struggling to negotiate the road back from brain trauma. Barton and Risker were both in the TLC program at the time *Broken Rhymes* was shot. Russell entered it later.

Along with providing continuing speech, occupational, psychological, and physical therapy, TLC teaches brain-injury victims how to make their beds, do their laundry, write checks and balance a checkbook, and all the myriad mundane tasks essential for independent living. Participants in the program begin in a group home, taking increasing responsibility for their own care and for such joint activities as preparing meals. For recreational therapy, they ride horses at Hope Arena, also established by the Moody Foundation. When they've mastered these and improved enough in emotional control and insight to function at a moderate level in the outside world, they move on to an apartment complex in which only some tenants are brain injured. They begin working twenty hours a week in low-stress jobs at American National Insurance Corporation (one of the Moody companies), the University of Texas Medical Branch, and other employers in the Galveston area.

After three years at Medical Center del Oro, Russell spent another three at the Transitional Learning Center. "In both places, I never saw anyone who was in a coma as long as myself," he later told the *Galveston Daily News,* using "coma" in its less precise, more popular sense to mean a persistent vegetative state. "It got kind of depressing watching people come and go." He added: "It's a lot of work going to TLC. But it's worth it. Every time I go there, I think that if it wasn't for TLC, I would be living in a nursing home."

Russell Moody made a remarkable recovery. Nine years after his accident, he was married and held a full-time job with his family's insurance company. But his speech remained halting, and he needed two canes to walk. Even his extraordinary persistence, his father's determined support, and the best rehabilitation therapy to be had anywhere in the world couldn't completely repair the damage inflicted in those brief seconds when he was catapulted 150 feet from his Jeep.

Most rehabilitation patients are not so fortunate. One of the major problems encountered by those seeking rehabilitation is the fragmentation of services. To achieve their full potential for recovery, people who have suffered serious brain injuries need physical therapy, speech therapy, cognitive retraining, occupational therapy, and professional help in dealing with emotional issues, sexuality, and social relationships. Assembling teams of professionals with equal skills in each of these areas is difficult. Brain-injury rehabilitation is a relatively new field, and there simply aren't enough trained and experienced people to go around. For example, a high percentage of victims of traumatic brain injury have difficulty speaking so that others can understand them. They must relearn not only word retrieval and organization, but also how to control breath, pace swallowing, and coordinate all the intricate muscle movements that allow us to form the sounds that make up words. That requires months and often years of work with a speech therapist. Yet the number of speech therapists in this country is severely limited. A for-profit group called Interspeech is attempting to fill this gap, but it provides only 6 percent of the speech therapists necessary to meet current needs. Because jobs in this field pay well, more young people are likely to seek training in speech therapy, but for the next several years, the demand for rehabilitation professionals will outstrip the supply.

Only a small fraction of the residual problems faced by brain-trauma victims are physical. The rest, the truly debilitating deficits, are mental and emotional. Some of these, such as memory loss, are obvious; others, such as social isolation, take their own insidious toll.

While some of the personality changes noted by therapists working with the brain-injured are directly due to physical damage to the brain, some—as seen in the film *Regarding Henry,* in which the character played by Harrison Ford is shot in the head and transformed from a nasty, aggressive lawyer into a nice guy—are a natural human response to the situation in which they find themselves. Those of us who have never awakened to find our once-whole bodies partially paralyzed or tried to communicate without being able to utter a word can only imagine how frightening and frustrating such experiences must be. Relearning functions we all take for granted can take months of exhausting work, and often these capabilities never return completely. Patients may begin to wonder whether the effort is worth it. No wonder they often explode in rage or sink into depression.

Such were the dilemmas encountered by Frederick R. Linge, a Canadian clinical psychologist who, at the age of thirty-nine and after sixteen years of practicing his profession, was in a disastrous head-on auto collision that left him with severe brain damage as well as a broken neck and numerous other fractures and internal injuries. Although doctors told his wife that he had little hope for survival, he gradually and painfully pulled his way back, eventually recovering well enough to function as a husband, a father, and a clinical psychologist. From the dual perspectives of a brain-trauma victim and a mental health practitioner, Linge wrote a revealing account of what it is like to suffer a severe brain injury.

Linge noted that, once he regained consciousness, one of his first challenges was becoming oriented: "During this period, I had no awareness of time. I existed in a world of the here and now. I was not even aware that such a concept as 'time' existed. I knew who

'I' was, but I did not think of myself as being a child, a boy, or a man. . . . One day, however, my 'mental clock' began ticking again and the concept of time began to become significant. . . . I began to orient myself in time, frequently becoming confused, but making steady progress. It was in the area of daily time that I first began to realize that I had a deficit within myself, since those around me were clear-headed and confident about the facts and I was not."

Even after making a remarkably full recovery, Linge was left without a sense of taste or smell and with short-term auditory and visual memory problems. He had developed a "one-track mind": he could focus with great persistence on a single line of thought, but if he were distracted, he would have trouble returning to it. And, not least important, he had a new personality.

> Having been a highly self-controlled person all my life, I found my-self with a hair-trigger temper and labile emotions. It is theorized that this state is due to CNS [central nervous system] irritation or else that some part of the brain, which is responsible for "braking" the mental motor, is dysfunctional after brain damage has occurred. . . . People close to me tell me that I am easier to live with and work with, now that I am not the highly self-controlled person that I used to be. My emotions are more openly displayed and more acces-sible, partially due to the brain damage which precludes any storing up of emotion, and partially due to the maturational aspects of this whole life-threatening experience. . . . My new openness of feeling makes it easier for me to communicate with others and for others to understand me.

For Linge, that release of the emotional brakes actually made his personal life more fulfilling and may even have helped him to relate better to his family, patients, and colleagues. But for people who are less tightly controlled before their traumatic brain injuries, this lessening of inhibition can be disastrous.

A few years ago, I received a call from a woman in West Virginia who asked for advice on dealing with her brain-injured daughter. Thanks to good luck and good care, the teenager had made an excellent physical recovery from her accident. She didn't look, sound, or move like a person who had suffered serious brain damage. But the injury had deprived her of both sexual inhibitions and judgment. Before the accident, the girl had been a normal adolescent, socially well-adjusted and appropriate. Now she was completely promiscuous and apparently oblivious to the potential consequences of her behavior. She would get into cars with complete strangers and consent to unprotected sex. Sometimes she would disappear for days. Her mother worried that she would become pregnant, contract the HIV virus, or be murdered by a sexual psychopath. The girl, however, seemed unaware that what she was doing was bizarre or self-destructive. She contended that she had recovered completely and was doing fine.

For brain-trauma patients who make what rehabilitation specialists consider moderate or good recoveries, physical problems such as partial paralysis or impaired eyesight represent perhaps 10 percent of their lingering disabilities. The rest of their deficits are cognitive and emotional. And for many, like the girl in West Virginia, the most difficult of these are flawed judgment and the inability to understand and acknowledge their remaining limitations.

Another such individual was Sara Burton. Before her accident, when she dozed off at the wheel of her car and drove into the back of a tractor-trailer truck, she was three months short of earning a master's degree in art therapy from Wright State University in Ohio. Despite severe brain trauma complicated by broken bones and internal injuries, Burton recovered her physical and cognitive abilities with remarkable speed. Nine months after the car wreck, she returned to school and began work on her thesis, which she recast in the first person and entitled "A Personal Therapy Process with Closed Head Injury: How it Feels to Be a Part of the Silent

Epidemic." Along with drawings that she had made during her rehabilitation, the thesis contained a heartfelt quatrain:

My name is Sara Burton.
For three months I've been hurtin'.
Will I ever be the same ol' me?
No one knows for certain.

By the time she received her master's, Burton thought she had in
fact become the same old her, but others didn't agree. After moving
to Dallas to be near her two older brothers, she found that she was
unable to land a job. Only when the Texas Rehabilitation Commission suggested that they place her as a client but not as an employee
did she confront the irritability and impulsiveness left as permanent
scars on her personality. "A lot of my sense was knocked out by that
injury," she admitted to Steve Blow of the *Dallas Morning News*.

Denial is one of the most common and pernicious effects of
traumatic brain injury. Such lack of insight causes particular problems when it comes to the operation of vehicles. If rehabilitation
goes well and the brain-trauma victim isn't left with serious physical, visual, or hearing damage, the time generally comes when he
or she feels ready to drive. For young people who were on their
own before their injuries and are now back living with their families, the thought of getting behind the wheel of a car or back on a
motorcycle often comes to symbolize independence and normalcy,
the first step in regaining their status as adults.

In reality, it should be one of the last steps. Driving an automobile and even riding a bicycle are much more complex and
potentially dangerous undertakings than our social practices reflect.
Either skill requires monitoring and analyzing numerous streams of
sensory data while both executing and coordinating precise physical maneuvers. With cars and trucks, we have at our command
tons of hurtling steel; one ill-timed move, one judgment error, and

we can wreak lethal destruction. With bikes and motorcycles, we may have less potential for inflicting injury on others, but—unprotected by passive restraints—we are terribly vulnerable to our own mistakes and those of the drivers around us.

One of the most common effects of even minor brain injury, the kind that doesn't require hospitalization, is difficulty handling complex tasks. Brain-trauma victims who resume driving or cycling are far more likely than other drivers to have accidents. Apart from being a threat to others, they are a particular menace to themselves. Reinjury is one of the prime causes of deterioration among people recovering from serious head trauma. The healing brain is incredibly fragile. A bump on the head or mild whiplash that would be insignificant in someone else can bring a promising recovery to a halt.

Although serious traumatic brain injuries cause the greatest problems for their victims, for their families, and for society at large, even minor head trauma can create significant difficulties. A bump that might not seem to warrant a trip to the hospital or a mild concussion that merits a few hours of emergency room observation, then release, can leave a person addled and irritable for weeks or even months. Pediatricians are beginning to recognize that some behavior and learning problems may have their root in a fall off a bike or a knock on the head—the sort of childhood mishap once assumed to be free of lasting consequences. The doctor examining an adult who has hit his head on a steering wheel during a parking-lot fender bender may warn him that he could experience problems keeping track of a busy work schedule or handling complex tasks.

Fortunately, individuals can compensate for these lingering effects, provided that they're told to expect them and are given techniques for dealing with them. A person used to relying on memory alone to keep track of meetings and assignments can start making lists and even can record conversations as a backup. If his stamina and ability to deal with stress have suffered, he can ask to have his workload reduced for a month or two. If he suspects that the injury has affected his judgment, he can postpone crucial decisions for a few weeks or consult trusted colleagues before taking action. The coping strategies that victims of severe brain trauma must use for the rest of their lives can keep minor head injuries from creating major havoc in careers and personal relationships.

Such strategies are one of the most promising areas of development in traumatic brain injury. As I mentioned in Chapter 3, research into drugs that may help repair damaged brain tissue or help the brain reroute functions once handled by cells now destroyed offers hope for the long term, but the less glamorous investigation of ways to help victims relearn the tasks of independence can improve their lives right now.

As with other aspects of health care, the most disenfranchised members of our society are also the ones who lack access to brain-injury rehabilitation. A disproportionate number of victims of brain trauma are uninsured. Males between the ages of fifteen and twenty-five make up the largest group of head-injury victims. Many of these, particularly those who suffer gunshot wounds, come from poor backgrounds. But even middle-class young men injured in car, motorcycle, and sports accidents are likely to be at the stage of life where their parents' insurance no longer covers them, yet they have little or none of their own.

Recovery from traumatic brain injury is often most rapid during the first year, because that's when the most active physical and neurological healing takes place. Regaining the skills needed to function in the world usually requires much longer. Doctors have learned not to mislead patients and their families into thinking that the process will be relatively rapid. The full course often takes ten years or more. Once the acute phase is past, rehabilitation is a lot closer to education than it is to medicine. Patients may have to relearn how to hold a spoon, how to speak, even how to control their anger. They may have to learn for the first time how to operate a wheelchair, walk with a cane, and keep lists as a backup for an unreliable short-term memory.

In our culture, we think of education as a phase of life, extending from childhood into our twenties and then stopping. But it's really a lifelong process—for all of us, but especially for those who've lost abilities to traumatic brain injury. While we place a high value on medicine, rewarding its practitioners with prosperity and esteem and investing billions a year in medical research and equipment, we undervalue education. That may be one reason that we have made far greater strides in the medical aspects of brain-injury treatment—our heroic rescues, high-tech imaging, state-of-the-art brain surgery, control of intracranial pressure and epileptic seizures—than we have in rehabilitation. When researchers find a new drug to limit secondary brain damage or announce that implanted cells may actually help devastated brain tissue regenerate, that's front-page news, partly because it is a medical breakthrough and partly because we want desperately to believe that there's a cure for every disease and disability, a cure just waiting to be discovered by science. If only the answer to the epidemic of traumatic brain injury were that simple.

We've also been far better at giving the head-injured access to medical care, regardless of ability to pay. By its very nature, brain trauma swiftly places its victims into the emergency medical system, from which they flow into acute care. Our society considers this kind of treatment a right—not quite like the right to free education from kindergarten through high school, since patients are responsible for their bills if they have insurance or assets, but if they're destitute, they are still supposed to get the same quality of care through the acute stage. Only when they are stable enough to be discharged from the hospital do inequities become blatant.

Although some regions of the country still lack sufficient numbers of rehabilitation facilities, the main obstacle keeping thousands of brain-trauma victims from reaching their full potential for recovery is money.

Because rehabilitation is largely education, providing universal access to such services does raise some knotty philosophical issues. Our society has agreed that we have a collective responsibility to rescue people from life-threatening situations; if they can't pay for the help, the bill gets shared by all of us, through taxes. But we haven't agreed to shoulder the collective cost of giving each individual the education that he or she needs to fulfill his or her personal potential. We stop at the twelfth grade; although states subsidize tuition at public universities, it isn't free. If we owe the brain-injured the education that they need to fulfill their potential, don't we owe all individuals the educations that they need to fulfill theirs?

Perhaps. But brain injury is a different case. Its catastrophic consequences often require us to offer special help to victims of traumatic brain injury. So does our enlightened self-interest. Although the day rate for an inpatient rehabilitation facility runs three to four times that for a nursing home specializing in head injuries, ten years invested in helping a brain-trauma victim recover enough to live independently and be self-supporting can save us fifty years of custodial care. Even if the damage is too great for that person to be able to make the transition from a life of total dependency to one of contribution, any substantial improvement can lower the cost that we will pay—either through taxes or through increases in our own insurance premiums—over his or her lifetime. Even if he or she remains too disabled to go out and get a job, an individual who can dress and feed himself or herself and help tend a communal garden in a group-living environment not only lives a richer, fuller life than one in a nursing home; his or her upkeep costs less.

In one sense, victims of traumatic brain injury never fully recover, because there is always permanent damage to the brain. I have no neurological or cognitive symptoms from my fall, but a piece of my skull is missing, and that makes my brain more vulnerable if I get hit on the same spot. As my brain ages, maybe I'll discover that I have a little less gray matter to spare than I would have had without that accident.

But even given the finest trauma and acute care and the best rehabilitation treatment available, many of the brain-injured go through the rest of their lives with significant deficits. Of patients who reach top-notch emergency rooms alive but with Glasgow Coma Scale scores of eight or less, 40 percent die, and 5 percent sink into a persistent vegetative state. About 10 percent end up severely disabled. Their physical and mental disabilities (usually both) are so bad that they need another person's help to perform such routine activities as eating, bathing, and dressing. Another 20 percent spend the rest of their lives moderately disabled, dealing with such obstacles as partial paralysis, memory deficits, and personality disorders. Given enough years of appropriate rehabilitation, close to half of these seriously brain-injured people make what neurologists and rehabilitation professionals call good recoveries. They can hold jobs and maintain interpersonal relationships. Even among these, a quarter suffer mild paralysis, a tenth reduced memory or intellectual abilities, and 17 percent epilepsy.

A good recovery in this sense may be a long way from a complete recovery. Take the case of James Blakely. He was working on a doctorate in education at the time he had his near-fatal car crash and suffered a closed head injury. Fortunately, he also worked for the Tucson public schools, so he had good insurance. Ironically, he taught students with learning disabilities.

For eighteen weeks, Blakely lay unconscious. Then he began the arduous journey through rehabilitation, employing some of the techniques that he had used with learning-disabled children. His judgment recovered less quickly than his cognitive abilities did. Three years after his accident, he called the police to report a lost cereal bowl.

After six years of rehabilitation, Blakely mastered a word-processing program on his home computer in preparation for a return to his doctoral studies. More than ever, he wanted to return to his teaching specialty, feeling that the insight and empathy he'd acquired at such cost would make him more effective. Because of damage to the part of his brain stem controlling balance, he still was confined to a wheelchair; he might never be able to walk. And he grieved over the stress and other burdens that his disabilities had placed on his wife and two young children. Yet by the standards of medical science, James Blakely was one of the ones who made what rehabilitation experts call a good recovery.

So was Gerard Papa. At eighteen, he graduated Phi Beta Kappa and summa cum laude from Columbia University, then went on to earn a law degree from Columbia in 1974. His senior year in law school, he started what was probably the first integrated basketball team in the racially torn neighborhood where he grew up — Brooklyn's Bensonhurst. After a stint with a Wall Street firm, he came back home to practice. When his Bensonhurst Flames captured the Brooklyn-Queens championship in 1981, they made the cover of *New York* magazine.

Five years later, in front of a Coney Island housing project, Papa and a friend were attacked by New York City policemen. Testifying afterward that they thought the two men were a pair of robbers that they'd been pursuing, the officers beat and kicked Papa with such force that he was left with permanent brain damage. By June 1991, the thirty-seven-year-old man, who had been the best student in his graduating class at one of the toughest universities in the country, could drive, but he couldn't practice law. He lived with his mother and spent his days running errands, visiting with friends, going to movies, and working with the Flames. He told the *New York Times* that he found himself pausing too long between phrases and had trouble connecting faces with names. "The zip," as he called it, was gone. "Imagine waking up tomorrow and having a different brain than you have today," he said. But by the standards of medical science, Gerard Papa had made a good recovery.

All our recent progress aside, we still haven't faced the toughest truth about traumatic brain injury: although the rhetoric of rehabilitation continues to focus on recovery and improvement, there are thousands and thousands of brain-injury survivors for whom recovery has peaked and any future improvement will be small. What do we do with the large population of chronically disabled brain injury victims who are not going to get much better, if at all? Once they've received all they can from rehabilitation, who will provide the support services that they need to function? At present, the burden falls on their families. But the challenge is greater than most families can cope with, and at the rate at which the epidemic is going, more and more will become overwhelmed by it.

Some brain-trauma victims bear a measure of responsibility for their injuries. They shouldn't have tried to drive after downing six beers; they should have worn a motorcycle helmet; they should have walked away from that fight. But in most cases, unless we dig deep for psychoanalytic explanations, we would have to say that the families of the brain-injured were innocent recipients of bad luck. Yet they often suffer as much as or even more than do the victims themselves. For the sakes of both the people who suffer traumatic brain injuries and their families, we need to develop better long-term solutions than those we have now.

· f i v e ·

How Families Become Victims

Jeff Davis and his wife, Susan Levine, had looked forward to escaping from Philadelphia's heat in August for a weekend in the Berkshire Mountains of western Massachusetts. Along with two other couples, they planned to bicycle the gentle hills and fields by day and catch pianist Emmanuel Ax's performance with the Boston Symphony at Tanglewood on Saturday evening.

On Saturday afternoon, Davis—a skilled, cautious, and knowledgeable cyclist (he was an associate technical editor at *Bicycling* magazine)—was riding his bike down a gravel back road. When his front bicycle tire hit an obstruction, he was thrown over the handlebars and landed on his head. If he hadn't been wearing a helmet, he almost certainly would have died. As it was, he suffered a severe closed head injury, shearing and stretching the axons that transmit nerve impulses to and from the brain. When he arrived at the Berkshire Medical Center, he scored only four or five points on the Glasgow Coma Scale. Davis was five weeks shy of his thirtieth birthday.

Thirteen days after the accident, when Davis was still in a deep coma, Levine used her American Express card to pay the $2,200 charge for the air ambulance flight from the Berkshires to the Hospital of the University of Pennsylvania in Philadelphia. It was another two weeks before Davis recognized her and spoke her name. Because he'd been careful (he'd worn a helmet) and lucky (the initial axonal damage was only moderate, and he'd received prompt, appropriate care to control pressure), Davis was able to leave the hospital just two months after his traumatic brain injury. His medical bill came to $78,007.15; fortunately, he had insurance to pay it.

More than six years later, Levine, a newspaper reporter, wrote an account of her husband's injury, describing what it was like to spend weeks wondering whether he would ever emerge from his coma. In one passage, she said: "Jeff's neurosurgeon, . . . with his team of residents and nurses, saved Jeff's life—his intelligence, his love of music, his generosity and spirit, his repertoire of bad jokes. In a different way, they also saved me."

Once Davis regained consciousness, Levine faced an unsettling uncertainty. Her husband was alive and alert, but was he the man she had married? Before the accident, Davis had been friendly and adaptable. Now, the staff at the rehabilitation hospital were describing him as defensive, disorganized, uncooperative, and lethargic. And Levine often caught the brunt of his personality change. "Once, as I pushed him to comply with some now-forgotten request, he asked my name," she recalled. "I told him and he replied, 'I have a wife named Susan, but she's nicer than you.'"

Fortunately, Davis made an almost full recovery. He emerged from rehabilitation with no lingering physical, cognitive, or speech defects, although he had become more cautious and had stopped riding bicycles. "There are no tears or anger anymore, only a kind of haunting sorrow for what was nearly lost," Levine concluded.

"We have different perspectives on that, of course. As Jeff tells me, 'You experienced it. I learned about it.'"

Levine suffered greatly with her husband—sometimes more than he did, since Davis was unconscious for weeks. Despite the months of agonizing uncertainty that she endured, despite the heartbreaking occasions when he didn't recognize her, Levine's story had a happy ending. The man she loved was restored to her.

Ardyce and James Masters weren't so fortunate. Their daughter Karen (not her real name) also suffered a traumatic brain injury, after which she was comatose for one week and semicomatose for one more—half the time that Jeff Davis was unconscious. Yet their experience was far worse than Susan Levine's.

Two months after Karen's near-fatal car accident in Oregon, the Masterses brought their daughter, who was then twenty years old, home to Montana. She had recovered most of her physical and cognitive capabilities, but her judgment and her ability to make decisions had been seriously impaired. Worst of all, she was emotionally unstable. As weeks passed, she became increasingly belligerent and suicidal. Alarmed, her parents turned for help to a local hospital, where the psychiatrist who treated Karen wouldn't even look at the medical records of her head trauma. Instead, he prescribed Haldol, an antipsychotic drug. Bouncing in and out of the hospital, Karen impressed some of the doctors who examined her as relatively normal, even fit to return to work. Head-trauma patients who have trouble curbing their angry or socially inappropriate impulses can often do so, albeit sometimes with great effort, in brief, structured situations. Dealing with people outside their families, they may appear to be perfectly normal for short periods of time; back at home or confronted with something irritating or unexpected, they may lose control.

Karen's doctors advised a three-month hospital stay to give them time to diagnose her problems and develop a plan to help her.

She refused and became completely uncooperative. As her mother explained: "Montana law makes involuntary hospitalization very difficult, so we waited helplessly until, angry because a local store refused to cash a check, she became violent and abusive. The police were called, and they took her to the hospital."

But Karen was very bright and verbal. At her commitment hearing, she persuaded the judge that she was being persecuted by her parents. After spending four months in a disastrous marriage to a man who had been a fellow patient at the hospital—an alcoholic more than twice her age—Karen killed herself. Nine years had passed since the accident that had left her intellect intact but her judgment and emotions devastated. Her mother's words reflect the helplessness and anguish experienced by so many family members of the brain-injured: "Over and over, her lack of judgment and capacity for forethought led her into desperate predicaments. Afterwards, she could see what she had done, and her self-hatred increased; but she could never seem to learn from her experiences. I cannot blame her for ending her suffering. . . . Her deficits . . . prevented the rational decision-making that would have allowed her to accept genuine help."

Most traumatic brain injuries shatter more than one life. Although one victim feels the physical impact of the fall, the blow, or the bullet, friends, colleagues, and especially family members feel its psychological impact. Tragedy ripples out to touch husbands and wives, parents and children. Virtually every case I've recounted in this book could be narrated either from the victim's point of view or from that of one or more significant family members who, in their own ways, were equally involved. This is true for my family as well as those of James Brady, Nancy Cruzan, Russell Moody, and many others.

Without adequate insurance, a settlement from a lawsuit, or other means for paying for appropriate rehabilitation, victims of traumatic brain injury, once they are medically stable, are usually transferred to a nursing home, where they receive little beyond custodial care. Often family members choose instead to bring the patient home, where they provide a better or at least more personal level of care. For severely disabled patients, this entails round-the-clock attention, usually on the part of a mother, wife, or daughter. If the caregiver had been working outside the home, the family suffers a drop in income. No matter what, the other family members are deprived of her time and nurturing. The family dynamic shifts not just to accommodate the brain-injury victim but to focus on him or her. Gone are vacations, picnics, and parties. Children feel uncomfortable bringing friends home.

Even when the money is available for appropriate rehabilitation, someone in the family may spend hours a day with the patient, reading aloud, praying, even becoming a kind of lay assistant in physical or speech therapy. To make this possible, the family may move in order to be closer to the institution. A mother who had previously juggled a full-time job with caring for four children may find her after-work hours devoted to caring for only one, leaving the responsibility for the others to her husband or her oldest daughter.

Whatever the victim's or family's resources, the time comes when most victims of traumatic brain injury go home. They may still be receiving speech and physical therapy, psychological counseling, and training in the skills of everyday life. These patients aren't ready to live by themselves, but they are ready to function outside an institutional setting.

The most obvious challenges to the household are physical and logistical. Doorways may need to be widened to accommodate a wheelchair. A bathroom may need to be added or remodeled. If everyone else in the family works or goes to school, schedules have to be rearranged or part-time help hired so that someone is always home with the brain-injured individual.

The Burke family's experience is typical. At seventeen, Lenny Burke ranked sixth in his high school class and had been accepted to two prestigious colleges when he was "submarined" during a basketball game. As he was poised in the air to make a lay-up shot, an opposing player hit his legs and catapulted him into a wild backward somersault. The right side of his head crashed onto the floor, propelled by the full force of his 6'1", 175-pound body.

Lenny spent forty-five days in a coma, another four and a half months in the hospital. After his release, his mother, Emmie Burke, later president of the Vermont Association of the Brain Injury Association, kept a log of his progress and of how the family adapted to living with the young man whose promising future had been destroyed. In an article offering practical advice to other families of brain-trauma victims, she wrote: "Lenny is the oldest of four children. When we brought him home, it was not only an adjustment for my husband and me, but for his brothers, Kevin (15) and Michael (13), and his sister, Kathy (11), as well. . . . At first, our younger children tried to adjust to Lenny's deficits, but after one and a half years, we found it much healthier for us all to expect Lenny to adjust to our family needs."

The Burke family developed a menu of techniques for establishing a realistic family routine and helping Lenny to adapt to it. Sharing these, Emmie Burke advised: make sure the injured family member showers, shampoos, and shaves every morning. If he has trouble dressing appropriately for the season, offer a choice of two outfits instead of giving him free rein to pick out his own clothes—and then sweat or shiver as a consequence of his impaired judgment. When he chatters on aimlessly or keeps repeating the same question or story, express your discomfort with the conversation, instead of saying something judgmental. Emmie Burke had a list of concrete, practical suggestions.

- Concentrate on all the positive progress.
- Discuss in detailed conversations with the injured person the many things that he or she *can* do.
- Write out positive phrases and place them in obvious places around the house (the refrigerator, the bathroom mirror, the wall of the family room).
- On a bulletin board, post some activity to look forward to each day.
- In the injured person's bedroom, hang a large calendar for keeping a schedule and crossing off each date at bedtime, and make sure that he or she carries a small appointment book during the day.
- Discuss articles in the daily newspaper, buy current magazines, and watch television news programs together.

Taken together, such accommodations represent significant time and effort by the family just to establish and maintain a semblance of normalcy. But these are minor inconveniences compared to the emotional challenges of living with someone who's suffered a traumatic brain injury. Recovery from acute brain injury—from the physical and medical consequences of the trauma and even from the damage to cognitive capabilities—doesn't mean recovery of personality. Especially in closed-head injuries, any patient who has been comatose for more than a few days almost certainly will suffer irreversible personality changes. They range from those as subtle as Jeff Davis's increased caution and slightly altered sense of humor to those as dramatic as Karen Masters's suicidal depression.

Even when clinicians try to communicate this information to families, family members often don't hear. Early on, they are so relieved that the person they love is alive and is regaining some capacity that they can't comprehend that full psychological recovery may never come. Later, when the victim looks and sounds like he or she did in the past, it is particularly difficult for families to revise the images and expectations that have sustained them. Just as brain-injury survivors often have extraordinary powers of denial, so do their families and friends.

For reasons that neuroscientists still don't understand, some of the most common and serious long-range problems suffered by the brain-injured are psychosocial. Study after study documents social isolation, lack of social contacts outside the immediate family, and socially inappropriate behavior even in patients who can walk and speak normally and who make the same scores on IQ tests as they did before their head trauma. It's easy to understand why a former athlete now confined to a wheelchair or a brilliant lawyer whose speech is now slurred might become depressed and irritable. Most of us can empathize when we read that former White House press secretary James Brady, a man famous for his sense of humor before and after the gunshot wound that almost killed him, slumped into depression when he recognized that he would never fully recover. In fact, some of the emotional problems experienced by the victims of traumatic brain injury are normal reactions to their conditions.

But in most cases, behavioral changes go beyond that. Some result directly from the battering of the brain; others are indirect consequences. According to neuropsychologist Muriel Lezak: "By and large, as the severity of the organic damage increases, the capacity for self-awareness, and particularly for accurate self-appreciation, decreases. Thus, the most profoundly impaired patients . . . are typically only dimly aware of their dysfunctions, if at all."

Because retraining the injured brain requires great concentration and effort, patients who are well enough to go through rehabilitation experience fatigue and frustration. Some of that response may be due directly to organic damage, some indirectly to an appreciation of how long and difficult the road ahead will be. But even people who suffer relatively mild concussions may experience fatigue for months afterward. They may start a two-hour project only to put it down after thirty minutes, to the inconvenience and annoyance of family members. Whatever the brain does that enables us to focus on a task and carry it through seems to be easily damaged even when most cognitive capabilities remain intact.

Brain-trauma victims also tend to have trouble assimilating new information and integrating it into their everyday behavior. Such learning difficulties also may make brain-trauma victims unaware of the social and judgment errors they make or, if they are aware, unable to stop repeating them. Imagine the frustration that a family member must struggle with in dealing with this day in and day out. A woman with a head-injured husband explained: "It takes him ten minutes to read a sentence, and a few minutes later he may not remember what he read. My husband has no long-term memory, and he can't follow directions. You tell him to turn off the light, [and] he'll shut the door."

Damage to brain tissue seems to heighten the anxiety arising from the patient's growing awareness of his disabilities. This can lead to paranoia, which may take forms ranging from suspicions about what family members are doing with the victim's money and belongings to intense sexual jealousy. A wife who has been faithful for years may have to face her head-injured husband's accusations that she's sneaking off to meet a lover whenever she leaves the house to go to the supermarket. Combined with the other stresses placed on the family, such behavior may eventually cause the very thing that the victim fears: it can drive the spouse away. Even without accusations to contend with, spouses of the brain-injured are often torn between guilt about wanting to abandon the injured partner and resentment at having to sacrifice so much of their own lives and satisfactions to care for someone who often doesn't appreciate the burdens undertaken on his or her behalf.

Many people who are brain-damaged display a childlike ego-centricity. They don't take into consideration the feelings of those around them. Perhaps because they have lost their own self-identity, victims of traumatic brain injury are often incapable of appreciating the needs of others. They may show a complete lack of gratitude for the enormous efforts and sacrifices that family members make on their behalf, and they may become unreasonably demanding, wanting every moment of the parent's or spouse's attention.

One of the most troubling results of head injury is a lack of impulse control, most commonly displayed as outbursts of anger. Sometimes a brain-trauma victim will hit, shove, or push. Such infantile physical battery, annoying in a three-year-old but potentially dangerous when delivered by someone with adult strength, tends to be directed far more often at family members than at strangers. Verbal diatribes are even more common, but such verbal abuse can sting as much as the physical variety, especially when it falls on someone who has devoted himself or herself to caring for the person who is lashing out. Children may not understand that the cause of their father's rage has little or nothing to do with their behavior or that his belittling stems from both his injury and his resulting competition for their mother's attention. Younger children may respond by developing learning and behavior problems of their own; older ones may escape by abusing alcohol or other drugs, developing other risky behaviors, or literally running away.

Victims of head injury may also become sexually promiscuous or crude, whatever their previous behavior or religious and cultural background. Sometimes internal restraints that prevent others from acting out certain thoughts disappear entirely. For example, one high school girl whose brother was injured in a motorcycle accident had to stop bringing her friends home because he invariably tried to kiss and fondle them.

The greatest challenge facing anyone close to someone who suffers a severe head injury can be accepting what has happened and the uncertainty of the outcome. Researchers who have studied the families of victims of traumatic brain injury have found that they react in stages similar to the famous five that Elisabeth Kübler-Ross identified as the steps people go through in confronting death and dying: shock and denial, anger, depression, bargaining, and acceptance. But for families of victims of traumatic brain injury, the stages of this mobile adjustment or process are different, and members may experience more than one at once or move back and forth among them, depending on how much or how little progress they see. The emotional road traveled by families of patients in persistent vegetative states includes grief and anxiety, guilt, denial, accommodation, and disengagement. With minor differences, most families of severely head-injured individuals pass over the same rough terrain. In some ways, reaching the point of accommodation may be even harder for the parents, spouses, siblings, and children of brain-trauma victims who make partial recoveries than for families of those in persistent vegetative states.

Lezak describes how a family's perceptions, expectations, and reactions to a brain-injured member develop over the course of two years. Initial happiness and relief that the patient is alive evolve into bewilderment when he or she doesn't act normally even three to six months after coming home. Families are prone to anticipate or at least hope for the victim's full recovery. When this doesn't happen, disappointment adds to the stress caused by the victim's troubling behavior.

Sometimes clinicians contribute to these problems by failing to adequately warn families that the brain-injured individual may emerge a very different person from who he or she was before the accident, even though that person may look the same and in many ways behave the same. Eventually, the family members become discouraged. They may become overwhelmed with guilt, blaming themselves for what they might or might not have done to prevent the injury. They may become depressed, feel trapped, or even fear that they might go crazy. The religious faith that brought them comfort and courage in the days immediately following the accident may become obsessive, or they may lose it altogether if they don't see the progress for which they've prayed so hard. If no one has explained to them that fatigue, irritability, angry outbursts, and lack of motivation are common, predictable results of traumatic brain injury, the family may come to perceive the victim as self-centered, irresponsible, and lazy. Not only do brain-trauma victims themselves need to be reeducated, but family members also have to be retrained in appropriate ways for communicating with and helping the head-injured person in their midst.

After a year or two of physical and cognitive recovery, many brain-injured patients become childlike and dependent. This is difficult for parents whose son or daughter may have just been entering adulthood at the time of the accident or assault. The work involved in rearing a child from infancy through adolescence makes it particularly difficult for parents to accept that their son or daughter may be stuck forever at some point in childhood, never regaining that recently won maturity and independence.

On excursions outside the house, there is always the risk of inappropriate behavior, ranging from poor bladder control to a tendency to shout rude or blunt remarks. Recounting her experiences living with her brain-injured stepson—a young elementary schoolteacher who suffered a closed-head injury in a car accident—Janette Moffatt Warrington described taking him out for a pizza between therapy sessions. David Warrington found the pizzeria's table too small for the pizza that they had ordered, so he simply pushed the table aside and proceeded to eat his pizza on the floor. David also had difficulty controlling his bladder, so if he happened to be somewhere that didn't have a bathroom when he needed one, he would simply urinate as he was walking.

The spouse of a head-trauma victim may experience a different but equally painful kind of distress. The injury may suddenly transform a person who before the injury was a companion and source of emotional and economic support into a lesser, often dependent role. Frederick Linge described his laborious attempts to fulfill a useful role in his family after the automobile crash that left his body shattered and his brain severely damaged: "As time went on and I grew stronger, I took over all of the housework, cooking, and cleaning, laundry, and so forth. I enjoyed doing these things, but at first they were quite an ordeal for the family. A shopping trip that would have taken my wife an hour would occupy an entire morning, with me making laborious lists, checking and rechecking, let alone the problem of getting me in and out of the car [and] maneuvering up and down the aisles with crutches, casts and shopping cart to be taken into account."

The marital burden multiplies because even when no physical impairments interfere, maintaining a satisfying sexual relationship can be extremely difficult. Some victims of traumatic brain injury lose all interest in sex, while others become obsessed with it and often behave inappropriately. One woman complained that her husband fondled her breasts every time she bent over to pour his coffee.

When a young child or an old man or woman suffers a severe head injury, the family sometimes finds adjustment somewhat easier. Even before such an accident, a toddler will have been dependent, with little judgment and undeveloped social skills; the emotional challenge for the parents will come in adjusting not so much to the child's situation shortly after the injury but to what may be limited prospects for the future. In many cases, people over seventy don't survive the sort of severe head trauma that leaves younger victims alive but impaired; when the elderly do survive, their families may have an easier time dealing with it because the families have already been mentally preparing for their care in their declining years.

Sometimes two sets of families or friends struggle over a victim of traumatic brain injury as if they were divorcing parents battling for child custody. When a 1983 car accident left her lover, Sharon Kowalski, brain-damaged and paralyzed, Karen Thompson fought for eight years to bring her back to their home. Denying that their daughter was a lesbian, Donald and Delia Kowalski placed her in a nursing home and refused Karen visitation rights. Finally, in 1991, Judge Robert Campbell stated that Sharon needed the companionship and support of both her families and designated a third party as her guardian.

From the best of motives, the family may become overly protective of its brain-damaged member. As he recovered his ability to function independently, Linge had to push his wife and children to stop treating him like a fragile invalid, behavior that impeded his progress. He explained: "At times I lost confidence in myself because they didn't think I could do something. This is a sensitive area and one that probably presents the greatest difficulty for the families of brain-damaged people. Most families have reserves of compassion and protectiveness that they can draw on in dealing with a hurt member. Supporting the injured one is not hard; it is the letting go that is difficult. It takes a great deal of sensitivity and courage for a family member to change roles at the appropriate time and let the handicapped person 'go it alone.'"

Some families are torn between becoming too possessive and controlling of their injured family member and their resentment that the injured person isn't able to be more independent. Others scapegoat brain-injured members, displacing anger onto them and blaming them for problems that have nothing to do with their disabilities. Long-dormant, unresolved emotional conflicts may come to the surface as the person with the brain injury attempts to regain lost capacities or to function in spite of disabilities. Similarly, family members may use the injured person's disabilities as an excuse for expressing feelings that had been held in check before the accident or right afterward, when the victim was at greater risk of serious disability or death. Such dysfunctional family dynamics not only increase tension; they can also prolong or derail the rehabilitative process.

Family problems surrounding brain injury naturally reflect the family's preexisting dynamics and relationships. If a family was well prepared to cope with an unexpected emergency, they may do better, at least initially, in coping with the brain injury. If a family was already on the brink of dissolution, the head injury may cause it to fragment. Some victims are already alienated from their families when their injury occurs, and the injury only exacerbates the alienation. Males in adolescence and their early twenties, who make up the largest group of the brain-injured, may be going through difficult or hostile separations from their parents. Alcoholics, whose drinking causes all too many car accidents, already have put other stresses on their families.

While some families fracture, others confronted with a similar emergency mobilize around it and pull together in order to care for an injured member. They may be able to draw inspiration and strength from religious beliefs or from supportive friends. Lenny Burke's younger brother, Michael, found his already close family drawn even closer by the tragedy. Analyzing the impact that Lenny's coma had on the Burkes, he wrote: "The month and a half that Lenny spent in a coma was the most trying experience my family and I had ever known. During those 45 days of uncertainty at the hospital, I came to know the great strength my parents possessed. . . . We all shared the same feeling of helplessness, and I believe it was this that brought us so close together as a family. We became open and honest in our communication with each other."

But no one is completely prepared for illness or disability, and we can't reasonably expect everyone to turn it into an opportunity for growth. Whatever growth occurs is only secondary to the suffering that has been endured.

One way that the Burkes were able to draw something positive from their tragedy was by helping others through their state's affiliate of the Brain Injury Association. Participation in brain-injury support groups helps many families cope. Even though the circumstances of the individual survivors and the individual families vary widely, people dealing with the vicissitudes of living with the brain-injured can give one another a kind of understanding that even the most empathic professionals cannot achieve. Such support groups have recently sprung up around the country, and both state organizations and the Brain Injury Association's central office in Washington, D.C., maintain directories of contacts.

No matter how positive an adjustment a family makes, each must deal with its own grief. Until a family understands and accepts the situation that they and their brain-damaged member face, they remain unable to mourn the loss of the person they knew and loved. Deprived of the comforting rituals that society has devised for mourning the death of someone close, they may have to create their own to mourn the loss of those parts of the personality that can't be regained. Ultimately, family members must detach themselves from their old expectations and form new ones based on the limited or altered capacities that their son or daughter, brother or sister, spouse or parent now possesses.

This task is difficult enough in itself. When limited economic resources and rehabilitation options force the family to choose between the welfare of the brain-trauma victim and the welfare of all its other members, too often the results are a shattered marriage, guilt-spawned depressions, and the loss of the potential contributions of three or four individuals, rather than one. Even when money isn't a problem, people who reach the fullest possible level of recovery from their traumatic brain injuries face a society ill-prepared to help them make use of their remaining capabilities—a society dependent on cars, short on empathy, and far less knowledgeable about traumatic brain injury and its individual manifestations than about AIDS or cancer.

We can do better, and we must. Fairness and compassion—two key values in our culture—require us to provide appropriate support to victims of traumatic brain injury and to their families.

Facing Fatality—and Worse Fates

Sometimes no rehabilitation is possible. Sometimes even the heroic efforts of the emergency rescue and trauma teams, the superb training and skill of the neurosurgeons, the tireless dedication of the acute-care staff, and the advantages of state-of-the-art technology are not enough. Each year in the United States, between twenty-eight thousand and forty thousand victims who survive to reach the hospital die later of their head injuries.

A conservative estimate that traumatic brain injury kills sixty thousand Americans annually means that even during a good year, it takes another life in this country every seven minutes. In the eleven years between 1981 and 1993, more Americans lost their lives to brain trauma than had died in all wars combined. And like war, it takes a disproportionate toll among the young. Even in this era of drug overdoses and the AIDS virus, traumatic brain injury remains America's leading killer of children and young adults.

In July 1989, Michael Doucette of Concord, New Hampshire,

won a nationwide contest aimed at identifying the safest teen driver in the country. The Dodge division of Chrysler Motor Company and AMVETS, a veterans group, sponsored Operation Driver Excellence, a competitive demonstration of automotive skill and judgment that Doucette described as "like a driver's test, only a lot harder." When Doucette won the contest, he was awarded a trophy, a five-thousand-dollar scholarship, and a year's use of a 1989 Dodge. In a tragic irony, this was the car that the seventeen-year-old boy was driving early one Friday evening the next February, when he was killed in a head-on collision. He apparently fell asleep at the wheel and drifted into oncoming traffic. Both Doucette and the other driver, nineteen-year-old Sharon Ann Link, were dead at the scene. As with most auto fatalities, the cause in both cases was traumatic brain injury.

Whether a brain-trauma victim dies at the scene, in the ambulance or helicopter, in the emergency room, or on the operating table, that death represents a life cut short, potential forfeited, contributions lost, and an intricate web of human relationships destroyed. Keen frustration, weary disappointment, and sometimes even nagging self-reproach can break through the wall of professional detachment to hit the doctors, nurses, and emergency medical technicians who work so hard to save the victim but fail. Family members and friends reel under the particularly devastating kind of shock and grief reserved for the survivors of those whose lives end suddenly, unexpectedly, and under violent circumstances.

No wonder hospital staffs go all out to save trauma victims. Physicians, nurses, support technicians—everyone working in emergency medicine—has been trained with lifesaving as an overriding goal. Our culture puts a huge investment, both technological and emotional, in rescue. Diagnostic procedures, surgical techniques, drug treatments, and monitoring systems all contribute to the team effort that may turn a catastrophe into a miracle. Whether we hear of them through factual news reports or see them in movies and soap operas, stories of such feats appeal to our romantic notions of being saved from danger and our yearning for instant gratification.

Our investment in rescue carries over to the attempt not only to save life but also to preserve and prolong it. After the initial efforts have succeeded, we don't want to lose the life that has been salvaged, so our acute hospital care also aims at keeping people alive with the assistance of advanced medical technology. This is all appropriate and worthwhile if we use our expertise and our technical resources to enable people to survive a crisis so they can be restored to normal or close-to-normal functioning. Individuals with what initially seem to be fatal injuries sometimes leave the hospital with capacities close to the those that they enjoyed before their accidents or assaults—with wounds, perhaps, but ones that will heal. That was my good fortune after my childhood fall. Even those who suffer permanent disabilities from their brain injuries may be spared more devastating damage thanks to proper acute treatment. The surgical, neurological, and supportive care that Russell Moody received prevented further complications from his accident.

Too often, however, our investment in rescue is combined with a lottery mentality. Once a life has been saved, we figure that as long as it is prolonged, there is always a chance, however remote, for recovery and restoration of function. This notion of beating the odds is a familiar feature of the American psychic landscape, and it helps to explain our fascination with such unexpected, unpredictable recoveries as that of Conly Holbrook.

On November 27, 1982, someone became murderously angry with eighteen-year-old Conly Holbrook. But instead of killing him, the assailant left the young North Carolina man severely brain-injured. For the first two months, he was completely unconscious, and doctors warned his family that he probably would die. For the next eight years, he sometimes seemed aware of his surroundings but spoke only in his sleep. His mother, Effie Holbrook, quit her job at a furniture factory and devoted herself to caring for him full-time. She underwent a revival of her lapsed Christian faith and prayed fervently for her son's recovery.

Then, more than eight years later, on February 25, 1991, while he was hospitalized during a bout with pneumonia, Conly spoke his first words: "Mama, I know who hurt me." Although his speech was halting and sometimes difficult to decipher, it was clear enough for his message to be understood: his cousin Donald Ray Combs was his attacker.

It was no accident that Conly Holbrook's story appeared in national newspapers on Easter Sunday. People who are given up for dead or "as good as dead" are occasionally resurrected. When this happens, and especially when the victim of traumatic brain injury not only survives but recovers, we all feel that the results were worth the enormous investment of time, resources, and effort. The problem is that all too often traumatic brain-injury victims survive but don't regain anything close to normal functioning. They are completely dependent on others for all their basic needs.

When a victim of traumatic brain injury dies, despite everything that dedicated caregivers aided by cutting-edge technology can do, the secondary victims—family and friends—begin to heal almost immediately. Our society has conventions and support structures to help them through this clearly defined grieving process. The family has a funeral to plan, thank-you notes to write for memorial contributions and flowers, belongings and assets to dispose of. Friends have pies and casseroles to bake and bring by, pleasant memories to share, sympathetic ears and shoulders to offer. Even when the death is a suicide, these rituals, formal and informal, impart a sense of closure. Each step makes it clearer that the head-trauma victim is irrevocably lost, at least in this life, to those who knew and loved him or her.

If the victim had health insurance, the insurance carrier pays the cost of the care that he or she received before dying. If not, the patient's estate may cover it, Medicare or Medicaid may pick up the bill, the family may pay, or the hospital writes off those thousands of dollars as uncollectible. Family members may require years of treatment for depression or other aftereffects of the emotional trauma, but the direct investment of time, money, and skill in caring for the victim ends when he or she is pronounced dead.

In the United States, most people who die of traumatic brain injury do so at the scene or within two hours of admission to the hospital. Of the patients who make it to emergency rooms, those with severe brain injuries—that is, those with scores of eight or fewer points on the Glasgow Coma Scale of fifteen points—about 36 percent die within a year and 53 percent regain some level of independent functioning. Around 8 percent return to consciousness but have such problems with memory, communication, thought processes, and impulse control that they require constant care for the rest of their lives. Another 3 percent, while physically alive, remain completely unconscious.

Technically, patients in this last group aren't in comas, although until recently doctors did lump them with the comatose. Someone in a true coma never opens his or her eyes, and a coma that lasts more than a few weeks is extremely rare. But each year traumatic brain injury leaves thousands (no one is sure exactly how many) in what now is called a persistent vegetative state (pvs). (Thousands more enter this limbo through drug and anesthesia overdoses, near drownings, and other insults causing severe shock or depriving the brain of oxygen.)

Because their brain stems survive the trauma relatively undamaged, patients in pvs breathe, their hearts beat, they perspire when they get too warm, and they shiver when they get too cold. They maintain a definite sleep-wake cycle, opening and closing their eyes at regular intervals. And because the brain stem regulates the alerting mechanism, they also open their eyes in response to painful pressure and loud noises.

Yet patients in a persistent vegetative state are far more profoundly unconscious than you and I are when we are asleep. Such people are alive only in the basic sense that their organs essential to passive survival still function. To all appearances, they have no awareness of surroundings, no fantasies or fears, no perception of pleasure or pain. When noxious stimuli cause their eyes to pop open, that's only a reflex. They are incapable of voluntary acts. Their biological tenacity is not a will to survive. They interact with no one; they share no feelings or thoughts, verbally or otherwise. Their bodies live, but their personalities are utterly absent. They are as cut off from family and friends as they would be if they were dead, yet our culture has no rituals for helping these loved ones acknowledge their loss and for comforting them in their grief.

Neurologists tread cautiously in diagnosing a patient as persistently vegetative. First, they rule out spinal injury or damage caused to the parts of the brain regulating speech and movement. In what's called locked-in syndrome, for example, a head-injury victim is aware of his or her surroundings but unable to talk or move his or her limbs when asked. Normally, however, the individual can blink one or both eyes in response.

Diana Dean lingered for a decade in what may have been locked-in syndrome. In March 1983, three months after she had graduated from a Dallas high school, she and her family went to Galveston for spring break. One afternoon at rush hour, at the busy intersection of two beach roads, a speeding pickup truck broadsided the car that she was driving. One of Diana's passengers, her sister Laura, suffered serious injuries but recovered fully; later she became an executive with the Brain Injury Association in Washington, D.C. The other passenger, Laura's best friend, Shanna Butler, died. After five weeks in acute care at the University of Texas Medical Branch in Galveston, ten months at Baylor University Medical Center in Dallas, a year at a rehabilitation hospital, and a total of $600,000 in medical bills, Diana reached the limit of her progress. She established a clear sleeping and waking cycle, and she seemed to have some awareness of what went on around her. The only way that she could communicate was to open one eye on command and use it to follow an object. As a way to wrest some meaning from their tragedy, in 1986 her family founded the Diana Dean Head Injury Guild, a nonprofit organization supporting head-injury prevention, education, and research.

Diana Dean was what neurologists call devastated; she was utterly helpless and would never recover the ability to talk, sit up, or clothe or feed herself. But if she was partially alert at least some of the time, she wasn't in a persistent vegetative state. Her family rearranged their lives and modified their home so that they could take care of her there. Ten years and four months after the accident, Diana died of complications from her injuries.

Because those who enter the hospital in a coma but later regain consciousness pass through a transitory vegetative state along the way, doctors classify patients as PVS only after prolonged unconsciousness, lack of response to verbal commands, and absence of any voluntary movements. By then, weeks have passed since the injury and subsequent surgery. Brain swelling and infection are under control. Without artificial hydration and nutrition (usually administered through a feeding tube), these patients would die within a few days; but with minimal attention to such basic needs, they could live for decades, especially if they are young and otherwise healthy.

Granted, even with everything modern medicine can do, chances are that these catastrophically brain-injured people will die. In a recent study of 650 head-injury patients brought into four university trauma centers and later diagnosed as persistently vegetative, only ninety-three—14.3 percent—were alive after six months. Of these, forty-seven regained some degree of consciousness by the end of the first year and another six did so by the end of the second. In other words, forty patients—close to half of the survivors—still lingered in a twilight zone between life and death. Alive but not living a life, they lacked the capacity for thought, feeling, or human interaction. Their lives consisted only of biological processes and reflex movements.

Persistently vegetative patients are medically stable but beyond the reach of medical therapy or cure. Very occasionally, someone who has remained in a persistent vegetative state for more than two years will show signs of responsiveness, but this happens in fewer than 1 percent of all cases. After someone has been unconscious for that long, many neurologists change the diagnosis of *persistent* vegetative state to a prognosis of *permanent* vegetative state. (To avoid confusion, in this book I use "pvs" only when I mean a vegetative state that is "persistent," not "permanent.") The dilemmas that this condition raises for individual clinicians, for families, for the health care system, for policy makers, and for our society as a whole are among the most perplexing we face today.

Take the famous case of Nancy Cruzan, who at the time of her accident was a vivacious young woman of twenty-six. On January 11, 1983, she was driving alone when she lost control of her car and crashed. Several minutes later, a passerby found her unconscious, lying facedown in a ditch, and not breathing. Emergency medical technicians resuscitated her at the scene, then rushed her to a nearby hospital, where she received trauma care. But because of the severity of her head injury and the length of time that her brain had been deprived of oxygen, her prognosis was grim.

For the first few weeks following her wreck, Cruzan seemed to be recovering. She was able to swallow and take food by mouth.

But then something happened to her brain—no one knows exactly what—and she deteriorated into a persistent vegetative state. She remained in this condition for four years while her family alternately hoped for a miracle and grieved over their loss. Gradually, they came to terms with the fact that her persistent vegetative state had become permanent. She was never going to regain consciousness, much less recover other capacities. Her parents eventually decided that the Nancy whom they knew and loved would not want to live in this limbo. As her guardians, they asked the nursing home taking care of her to stop the artificial feedings that kept their daughter—or at least her body—alive. When the nursing home refused their request, they went to court.

The judge agreed that Nancy Cruzan's parents had the authority to make this demand on behalf of their daughter, but the nursing home remained adamant, setting in motion a legal wrangle that went all the way to the Supreme Court. For the first time in its history, the nation's highest judicial body ruled on a "right to die" case. In a long and complicated set of opinions, the justices struggled to find adequate words to capture and address the many troubling and subtle issues raised by the Cruzan case. The court indicated that individuals have a constitutionally protected "liberty interest" in accepting or refusing medical care, including such life-sustaining procedures as intravenous hydration, artificial feeding, and mechanically assisted respiration. But the court also ruled that states have the authority to demand high standards of evidence about how patients, before they were injured, said they wanted to be treated if they ever fell into a permanent vegetative state.

Armed with the Supreme Court's decision, Cruzan's parents returned to the court where they had filed their original petition. Once again, bolstered by additional testimony about her general attitude and specific preferences, which suggested that Cruzan would not want to be kept alive in a permanently unconscious state, the local court ruled that the parents had the legal authority to insist on her behalf that the artificial feeding be stopped. The nursing home complied. In a few days, Cruzan died. More than four years had passed since her parents had filed their first petition, more than eight since her accident.

Numerous surveys reveal that 90 percent of Americans would not want their organic life prolonged if they were permanently unconscious. Many say that they consider a permanent vegetative state a fate worse than death. As far as we can tell, for the patient, it is a fate equal to death, because he or she doesn't cognitively experience anything. For the family, however, losing a loved one to a permanent vegetative state almost certainly is worse than losing him or her to unambiguous, organic death. The moral and financial burden of seeing that the shell of that person receives adequate care continues. There is no closure, no ritualized comfort for grief.

Yet, surprisingly, family members are often reluctant to "pull the plug" and terminate life support, even when assured that this is legally and ethically permissible. Those closest to the patient may never give up hope or may hold out for a miracle, even if reason tells them that the chances for one are infinitesimally remote. Although Conly Holbrook spent eight years too devastated to speak, he wasn't completely unconscious; even his seemingly miraculous recovery wasn't a return from a permanent vegetative state.

For fear of appearing to be insensitive or, worse still, advocates for euthanasia, doctors and hospitals are reluctant to challenge families clinging tenaciously to hope even if they disagree with them. Complicating the issue on every side is our collective confusion about death. As a culture, we have difficulty facing fatality. On one hand, we see it every day. Local television newscasts lead their nightly programs with murders, lethal industrial accidents, and multifatality car wrecks. Network broadcasts take us live to the site of the latest global catastrophe, showing us the bodies of fellow human beings killed by war, famine, earthquake, or epidemic. Action-adventure films rack up staggering body counts on the way to setting records at the box office. Yet as a society we do not accept death as a natural end to life. Instead, we suffer from a Ponce de Leon complex, always in quest of the fountain of youth, the cure for disease, the wonder drug or therapy that will restore function. We distance ourselves from personal contact with the dead and dying. Nowadays, despite the increasing popularity of in-home care for the terminally ill, most Americans still take their last breaths in hospitals, many in intensive care units—one of the most alienating and artificial environments imaginable.

We find it especially difficult to accept the deaths of people who die unexpectedly from accident or violence or who die young, long before their time. Since most victims of traumatic brain injury fall into both these categories, we're reluctant to give up on them. The present high-tech trauma care in place at major hospitals across the country is superbly suited to saving the lives of victims of severe head trauma. It does an outstanding job of snatching them back from sudden and untimely death. But the heroic urge to rescue, so fitting for emergency situations, exerts a prolonged influence in our health care system. Aggressive intervention to save the lives of trauma victims is often followed by stubborn resistance to withdrawing care, even when it is obvious that the continuation of life-sustaining procedures is futile. Once we've initiated rescue in a medical setting, we seem unable to stop. When a hiker is lost in the wilderness or a sailor is lost at sea, eventually we give up the search. But having pulled a trauma victim back from the brink of death, we seem unable to accept the fact that our medical system may not be able to help that person resume any but the most technical semblance of a life.

One reason for this reluctance is our psychological investment in the patient. To the emergency medical technicians, the neurosurgeon, and the acute-care nurses, the patient's survival represents enormous effort, the intense focus of their training, experience, and dedication. To the family, the fact that the patient is alive means that he or she has already beaten the odds. If the doctors were wrong about that person's dying, they might also be wrong about his or her chances of recovering consciousness and function. After all, *Sleeping Beauty* is one of our favorite fairy tales.

Our culture evinces a strong current of vitalism—the value system that holds that any human life is precious and should be biologically prolonged as long as possible and at any cost. Only a small minority of Americans actually subscribe to vitalist principles when it comes to how they wish to be treated, yet this perspective has a pervasive influence on how we treat the catastrophically injured. The goal of saving and preserving life is deeply rooted in Western medical tradition, and hospitals and health care professionals often allow this goal to override all other considerations.

On top of this, hospital administrators and health care professionals often mistakenly fear that failure to do everything possible to preserve life renders them vulnerable to legal liability or bad publicity. In addition, they may have a vested economic interest in prolonging the lives of patients, even the permanently unconscious. As long as someone pays—Medicare, Medicaid, a private insurance carrier, or the patient's family—all the financial incentives favor continuing artificial life support. Even doctors who object to using futile life-extending technologies operate in an environment increasingly driven by economic considerations.

As a cornerstone of medical ethics, respect for personal preferences can overcome the pressure to keep the permanently unconscious patient organically alive for years and even decades. But most victims of traumatic brain injury are young and healthy, not the sort to have drafted the advance directives that are popularly called living wills. Without such documented preferences concerning artificial life support, physicians and hospitals usually do nothing to hasten death unless clearly authorized by a guardian or a court to do so.

This is nothing new. In his 1992 memoir *Down from Troy: A Doctor Comes of Age,* author and retired surgeon Richard Selzer describes a scene that had taken place about fifteen years earlier, when he and the house staff were making rounds in the new trauma unit of a major hospital in Pittsburgh. He says the patients were mostly men and women who had been in auto accidents, with two exceptions. The first of these was a young gymnast who had miscalculated a tumble and was now quadriplegic. Selzer continues:

> In the next bed was a young farmer who had been struck on the head by a falling tree. Such an event could have taken place in prehistoric times. His electroencephalograph was flat. There was no hope of his waking up. Every four hours the resident doctors inserted a tube into his lungs to suction away the secretions, feeding misfortune that it might endure.
>
> "At what point," I asked them, "will you stop thinking of pneumonia as an enemy?"
>
> "That is a philosophical question," the resident told me. "I don't deal with them."
>
> "If he were your brother?" The young doctor murmured something and looked down at his shoes.

Permanently unconscious patients often linger in their limbo for years, surviving with the assistance of artificial feeding and routine nursing care until they die of infectious disease or a condition related to their initial injuries or subsequent inactivity. If they were strong and healthy before their accident or assault, they may survive to within a decade or two of their normal life expectancy.

Meanwhile, families adapt in their own ways. Some abandon their permanently vegetative relative to institutional caregivers and get on with their lives. Others regularly assist with the nursing or provide the care at home. A few families, like the Cruzans, do seek legal authority to stop artificial life support or negotiate with the caregivers to do so. Thanks to the legal battle sustained by Nancy Cruzan's parents, such families' ordeals have generally become less grueling.

Once patients have been reliably diagnosed as permanently vegetative, no one is quite sure what to do for them. On one hand, physicians can sustain the organic lives of such patients for days, months, or years. Yet no other medical goals can be achieved. These patients cannot be cured; they cannot be restored to consciousness. Some argue that keeping permanently vegetative patients alive is a misuse of precious resources, because these patients have no prospect of recovery. Yet these totally dependent individuals are the most vulnerable people in our society. And one of the primary goals of any advanced civilization is to protect the vulnerable.

Ambiguity extends and often intensifies the sadness and suffering of each patient's family and friends. Some cling to a thin thread of hope for a miracle, even after years pass. Others take refuge in denial, insisting that reflexes such as swallowing or random arm movements are a sign of subjective awareness.

The clinical dilemmas raised by permanent vegetative states would be so much simpler if neurologists could tell in the trauma center or operating room which victims of traumatic brain injury would become permanently vegetative. The medical community could simply agree that artificial nutrition and hydration were not appropriate treatments for these patients. By never ordering that a feeding tube be inserted, doctors would spare themselves the dilemma of whether and when to remove it.

But our diagnostic technology cannot predict at the time of injury which brain-trauma patients will die, which will be permanently vegetative, which will be conscious but severely disabled, and which, given good luck and appropriate rehabilitation, will make fairly full recoveries. To give these last two groups a chance, the acute-care team has to do everything in its power to keep all four groups alive. We can't foist off on them our collective responsibility for confronting the issues raised by those who linger in vegetative states.

The longer a patient spends in a persistent vegetative state, the more unlikely it is that he or she will ever recover even minimal consciousness. After two years, even the most conservative neurologist would change the diagnosis of persistent to a prognosis of permanent vegetative state. Once this grim verdict is reliably rendered, both reason and compassion tell us that all forms of medical treatment, being futile, should cease. Nature should be allowed to finish what accident or assault started. The family should be allowed to grieve and be comforted.

Still, what about the feeding tube that has kept the vegetative patient alive throughout those two years? What about the doctor who orders it removed and the nurse who carries out these orders?

Clearly, stopping life-sustaining procedures for a patient who otherwise is not dying causes his or her death. Without an advance directive from that individual or the orders of a legally authorized representative acting on his or her behalf, this is arguably euthanasia. Some physicians, bioethicists, and policy makers seek to finesse the ambiguity of PVS by arguing that once patients are determined to be permanently unconscious, they should be declared dead.

But passage of time is the only way to know that someone is permanently unconscious. We can be virtually certain that a person who has remained in a persistent vegetative state for a year will never recover awareness; once two years have passed, the chance of that individual regaining even the most basic level of consciousness is minuscule. Yet setting such calendar limits would put us in the position of saying that a patient who was alive on Tuesday was dead on Wednesday, even though his or her objective status was unchanged. When it comes to the permanently vegetative, the line between life and death is blurry; we can't make it more distinct by fiat.

Permanently unconscious patients are not, by our usual criteria, dead. They breathe, often on their own, and their hearts beat without mechanical assistance. Their brain stems are able to maintain blood circulation sufficient to keep their vital organs operating. For all meaningful purposes, their personal history may be over, but they are not brain-dead.

After years of grappling with this enigma, I have concluded that while this may be life, it is not human life. Merely the organic functioning of our bodies doesn't constitute being human. Being persons requires having a personality, being aware of our selves and our surroundings, and possessing human capacities, such as memory, emotions, and the ability to communicate and interact with other people. These ingredients of our humanity may be damaged or limited—some may even be lost—without forfeiting our claim to personhood. But when they are all totally absent, forever and irrevocably, as is the case with the permanently unconscious, we are no longer human beings; hence society no longer has a moral responsibility to sustain our lives. A physician who orders a stop to artificial feeding and hydration in such a case ends a life, but only an organic life. He or she doesn't commit murder.

I recognize that from the standpoint of bioethics and of law, this is shaky ground indeed. We don't know what to do with patients in permanent vegetative states because we don't know what to say about them. Are they alive or dead? Persons or nonpersons? One thing is certain: they are wholly vulnerable, totally dependent on our willingness to provide the essentials of life, such as food and water. If we discontinue nutrition and hydration, they will die. We try to make such a decision tolerable by emphasizing that the nutrition and hydration are "artificial." But we can't get around the fact that they are hardly more so than feeding an infant with a bottle, and they certainly rely more on labor than on technology.

With our constant but routine and low-tech help, permanently vegetative patients may survive for decades. If we stop feeding them and giving them water, they will die within days or at most weeks. Because they are totally unconscious, this death will not be painful; nonetheless, it will be certain. Even if our primary motive is to discontinue futile treatment—a valid medical decision—rather than to cause their death, we know that they will die as a result of our actions. That makes it hard to dodge the charge that this is a form of euthanasia: causing the death of a patient who would not die were the current treatment to continue.

The key to this dilemma lies in current hospital policies. As matters now stand, unconscious patients are assumed to want their lives prolonged artificially, whatever the prognosis, unless they have left clear evidence to the contrary. In other words, the burden of proof lies with the family seeking to remove artificial life support.

In Philadelphia, Joey Fiori lingered in a vegetative state for twenty-four years. In 1971, ten days before he was to marry his childhood sweetheart, the young Vietnam veteran had a motorcycle accident that left him severely brain damaged. Before the wreck, Fiori, who had scored 147 on an IQ test, had hoped to become a career navy officer specializing in nuclear physics. After more than a year of rehabilitation, the best he could do intellectually was to play simple card games. His speech consisted of two words: "I" and "itch."

In 1976, Fiori suffered an epileptic seizure brought on when a local Veterans Administration hospital failed to medicate him properly. The seizure threw him into a permanent vegetative state. Admitting their ultimate responsibility for the medical malpractice, the federal government paid for his care at Philadelphia's Mayo

Nursing Home, which cost $150,000 a year. But the emotional burden fell on Fiori's mother, Rosemarie Sherman, who brought friends together for bedside prayer vigils. In 1992, realizing that her son would never regain consciousness, she asked the nursing home to remove his feeding tube. It refused to do so without a court order.

Like the overwhelming majority of twenty-one-year-olds, Joey Fiori hadn't left a formal advance directive or even letters or diaries expressing in writing what his desires were should such a decision ever need to be made. Because he had served in Vietnam, surely he must have faced the specter of his own death, but he may not have considered the possibility of survival without thought, emotion, or awareness.

Fiori's lack of a clear statement about his wishes should he ever lapse into a PVS created a legal nightmare as the state and the courts grappled with determining who could make decisions in his place and what decisions could be made. However, in January 1995, in the midst of the motions, hearings, and appeals, Fiori died of pneumonia. As an ironic ending to this tragic story, a year after his death and three years after his mother had first requested that his feeding tube be removed, the Pennsylvania Supreme Court finally held that Rosemarie Sherman may, without court involvement, have the life-sustaining treatment removed from her son if two physicians consented. For Fiori, of course, this was too little, too late. Let us hope that other families may be spared similar ordeals.

How much more humane it would be for Rosemarie Sherman and thousands of others in her situation if we assumed, consistent with the wishes of nine out of ten Americans surveyed, that no one would prefer a life of permanent unconsciousness sustained and extended by such technologies as feeding tubes. This new presumption should be announced clearly in legal statutes and hospital policies, and it should be communicated to the public, so that those who would want to be kept alive under those conditions can draft advance directives stating so.

Of course, patients who have expressed a preference for being kept alive in PVS experience no satisfaction from their choice once they become permanently unconscious. Their families endure but are unlikely to welcome the role of caretaker for an individual who isn't even aware of their presence, let alone the sacrifices that they are making. Even if money is available to pay for the care, there is something ethically repugnant about the futile expenditure of limited economic and professional resources.

But tolerance of diversity is one of our culture's most important values. To uphold it, we must allow vitalists to seek life at all costs. That doesn't mean that they should be entitled to receive it upon demand. They should have to arrange to pay for extending their lives in such circumstances, and insurers might soon discover the profit potential in offering separate policies covering permanent vegetative states. Since the actuarial chances of any one individual being rendered permanently vegetative are slim, insurance premiums could be affordable; they might even incorporate a modest surcharge to go toward insuring vitalists who are indigent.

The state should regard vitalism as a personal and private matter, like religious education. While our shared values demand that we respect the views of vitalists, their values do not impel us to support them with public funds. Spending millions or even thousands of dollars to sustain the mere biological existence of patients who will never recover consciousness is not just futile; it is also unfair to the victims of traumatic brain injury whom that money could help, including those who are only passing through the limbo of a persistent vegetative state.

Protecting the Most Vulnerable

Before 1990, the biggest obstacle faced by victims of traumatic brain injury was the lack of rehabilitation facilities focusing more on education and training than on medicine. Although the United States still does not have all the rehabilitation centers that it needs, the number of these facilities has tripled in the past decade. Overall, this is good news for brain-trauma patients and their families. But such explosive growth also sounds a warning for those of us concerned with health care policy, either directly as practitioners and lawmakers or indirectly as consumers and taxpayers. The same profit motive that fuels the rapid response to real needs can also lead to misrepresentation, inflated charges, patient abuse, and outright fraud. These pitfalls plague the entire health care industry, but because the brain-injured are so vulnerable, we have an added responsibility for protecting them from exploitation.

In 1987 I obtained an advisory memo put out by the San Francisco investment banking firm of Robertson, Colman, and Stephens. Under the title "Traumatic Brain Injury: The Most Dynamic Niche of the Medical Rehabilitation Industry," it included then-current versions of many of the troubling statistics that I've cited in this book. But the conclusion was that the epidemic presented an excellent opportunity for making money. The report stated candidly, "We believe head-trauma rehabilitation has outstanding growth potential, with projected revenues exceeding $3 billion by 1992."

Offering an impressively cogent and concise analysis of traumatic brain-injury rehabilitation as a business, Robertson, Colman, and Stephens parsed the industry into four main types of facilities:

- Coma-treatment programs offered in acute-care hospitals, rehabilitation hospitals, and skilled nursing facilities (SNFs).
- Post-acute-care intensive rehabilitation programs offered in rehabilitation hospitals and SNFs.
- Transitional living programs offered on an outpatient and inpatient basis.
- Independent living, an informal program in which patients receive various therapies in outpatient settings. Residents live either in a group house setting or in a totally independent setting.

Calling the cost of brain-injury rehabilitation services "tremendous," the white paper noted that treatment costs from $1,000 to $2,000 per day in an acute-care hospital and from $350 to $1,000 per day in a post-acute-care rehabilitation hospital. The investment bankers found that skilled nursing facilities dedicated to the brain-damaged charged from $7,500 to $18,000 a month, that transitional living programs averaged $10,000 a month, and that day treatment centers and life-long residential programs for the brain-injured averaged $3,000 a month.

As I read the figures that Robertson, Colman, and Stephens had assembled, I realized that with medical costs skyrocketing at twice the general rate of inflation, these fees might easily double within ten years. The investment bankers went on to explain that as the industry grew, it was becoming increasingly concentrated. Almost one-third of its income, 32 percent, was brought in by six corporations, which generated combined annual revenues of $184 million from brain-trauma rehabilitation. A handful of not-for-profit rehabilitation hospitals produced another $5 million. The remaining $391 million was scattered among more than four hundred smaller providers.

Robertson, Colman, and Stephens identified four among the six emerging rehabilitation giants as having particular promise for profit. One was a company called New Medico, which the summary described as having "five transitional living facilities and a number of coma-treatment programs in its skilled nursing facilities." The report added: "New Medico's transitional living programs differ from the transitional living programs offered by most other companies in that they are in isolated rural areas and serve large populations of 100–200 patients. Most other transitional living programs are small (10–35 patients), community-based programs."

Five years later, New Medico's name came to my attention again. Just as the investment wizards had predicted, the Lynn, Massachusetts, company had grown. It now operated thirty-six rehabilitation centers in fifteen states. And it was a target of two congressional subcommittees: Ted Weiss's Human Resources Subcommittee of the House Government Operations Committee and Ron Wyden's Subcommittee on Regulation, Business Opportunities, and Energy, which, according to the *New York Times*, was investigating what Oregon congressman Wyden called "waste, fraud, and abuse in this rapidly expanding field of health care."

Health care in America has always been plagued by fraud, abuse, and false promises. From nineteenth-century patent medicines to the herbal cancer cures touted in today's tabloids, needy and vulnerable individuals have always made tempting targets for unscrupulous entrepreneurs. In the late 1980s and early 1990s, the high-profile scandals involving private psychiatric hospitals were only chapters in a continuing saga.

Although complaints poured in about other brain-trauma rehabilitation companies, New Medico received a disproportionate number. A *New York Times* article written by Peter Kerr and reporting on the subcommittees' work described the company as having been founded in 1982 by Charles Brennick, who had owned a nursing home. Brennick lacked any formal training in rehabilitation. In fact, he hadn't finished high school. But he was regarded as an astute businessman, and he had several sons to help him expand and run the company.

Reckoning that brain-injury rehabilitation represented more than three times what Robertson, Colman, and Stephens had predicted—$10 billion in gross annual revenues, most paid to multistate, for-profit providers—the Wyden subcommittee heard allegation after allegation of cruel and inhumane treatment; exploitative, inappropriate, or illegal billing practices; questionable treatment choices driven by benefit coverage rather than appropriateness; and aggressive, unethical marketing practices.

Therapists reported being fired for refusing to falsify patient records to show that patients were making progress when they weren't. Staff told of being pressed to keep patients as long as possible, provided that they had the means to pay, but to dump patients once their insurance ran out. One referral coordinator described being directed to call a patient's family and say that the doctor had recommended one of New Medico's facilities, then call the doctor and say that the family had chosen New Medico.

Spokespeople and lawyers for New Medico and the other publicly traded brain-injury providers dismissed the allegations as the unfounded complaints of disgruntled former employees and of patients' families with unrealistic expectations. Any problems that did exist, they insisted, had been corrected.

In a separate probe conducted by a subcommittee of the Texas state senate, a brain-injury patient named Jim Hudson told of his experience in New Medico's rehabilitation facility in Tyler, Texas, in 1991. Then fifty-six years old, he was eager to return to work, and, as he told Mark Smith of the *Houston Chronicle,* New Medico told him that their program would enable him to do so. He traveled to Tyler for what he understood would be a two-day visit, during which he didn't see any doctors or observe or participate in any therapy sessions. When he advised the staff that he had decided to leave, they told him that he had signed papers that prevented him from doing so. As the *Chronicle* related his story, "Hudson called his wife and an attorney, but said when he tried to walk out of the building, he was surrounded by a marketing staffer and two security guards brandishing night sticks." After a forty-five-minute standoff, Hudson said, he walked away from them to use the bathroom and realized that his wife was sitting in a van in front of the facility. He quickly walked out and into the waiting vehicle.

Patient advocate Lucy Gwin, who spent three weeks in 1991 as a patient in a New Medico facility in Cortland, New York, described seeing her roommate being raped at least twice by a staff member. The roommate's brain embolism left her unable to talk, but she was conscious, and she could cry. When Gwin tried to stop the second rape, the man and the two friends who were helping him pushed her down a flight of stairs. She reported the rapes to the New York State attorney general's office, but an investigator told her that she wouldn't make a credible witness because she was brain-damaged.

Because confusion and paranoia are common long-term effects of severe brain trauma (recall James Blakely, described in Chapter 4, who reported his lost cereal bowl to the police), patients complaining of mistreatment often encounter officials' disbelief.

This is all the more reason for us to put in place regulations for assuring that the staff at rehabilitation facilities are carefully selected, well trained, and closely supervised.

The congressional subcommittees heard even more appalling stories on neglectful treatment or outright abuse at for-profit rehabilitation centers.

> Mr. A, a twenty-two-year-old automobile accident survivor, was placed in an out-of-state facility while still in a coma. When he revived, he was hard to manage, manifesting behavioral problems demonstrated by many brain-injured people. Staff at the for-profit facility locked him in a coffinlike box.

> Ms. G, a twenty-two-year-old saleswoman who had been brain-injured in an accident, was transferred from a rehabilitation center to a lock-up facility within the same organization. The move was challenged by her parents, and the company discharged Ms. G to a state facility for the mentally ill. The parents got her transferred to another provider of rehabilitation services, who weaned her from a heavy, "therapeutic" drug regimen begun during her initial rehabilitation commitment. Within nine months Ms. G was discharged. She now lives independently, has a job, and is going to school.

> Massachusetts authorities report that last summer, a brain-injured patient at a for-profit rehabilitation center was killed by an accidental overdose of morphine, and another patient had to be revived after air from a breathing tube was cut off.

A mother described visiting her five-year-old son at New Medico's Slidell, Louisiana, facility and finding feces in his bed and black mold on his blanket. Although neglect like this also happens in poorly run nursing homes and even acute-care hospitals, this woman thought that she had chosen a top-rate rehabilitation center. She had sent the boy to this particular place after being told that its coma program, which included playing music for patients and talking to them, could help bring her son out of his persistent vegetative state.

In his testimony before the Wyden subcommittee, Nathan Zasler, director of the brain-injury research center at the Medical College of Virginia, questioned the efficacy of such "coma stimulation" techniques as reading newspapers to deeply unconscious patients. Although they constitute a staple on the menu of services provided by coma treatment centers, studies have yet to demonstrate that they do anything to improve outcome. Yet the providers bill these treatments out at hundreds of dollars per hour. "I don't feel ethically it's something I should be charging the payer or family for," Dr. Zasler told the subcommittee.

Former professional staff and families of patients reported case after case in which services, proven effective or not, were promised but never delivered. And the profit leaders in the industry spend plenty on making those promises. When I've attended national conferences on head injuries, I've been struck by how rehabilitation centers promote themselves. Their brochures incorporate award-quality graphics featuring four-color photos of appealing patients and families working with caring and competent staff to restore the head-injured person to normal life. She may be in a wheelchair, but she's applying eye makeup and operating a computer. He may use a walker, but he's standing up and throwing a football. The building, grounds, and interior decor are worthy of a Hyatt hotel.

Testimony in the congressional hearings described how public relations and marketing specialists employ sophisticated techniques designed to exert an irresistible emotional appeal on families at their most vulnerable. In many facilities, a staff member combs the daily newspapers, looking for reports of auto accidents and assaults involving brain injuries. Then someone is assigned to contact the family while the patient is still in the acute-care hospital.

From a nurse who had worked for both acute-care hospitals and for-profit rehabilitation companies, the Wyden subcommittee learned that multistate brain-injury rehabilitation chains have salespeople who "make the rounds, in some hospitals, with doctors and nurses in the ICU." She added that the rehabilitation representatives buy meals for hospital staff and that "they fly physicians, nurses, and [hospital] social workers around the country to show off facilities."

Families also reported being offered expense-paid trips to check out rehabilitation centers. The subcommittee report went on to say: "Parents and guardians told subcommittee staff stories of being waylaid at the hospital by representatives of rehab providers, and of being 'wined and dined' by those representatives in order to get their referral. Subcommittee staff also were told that some staff at acute-care hospitals were on informal 'commission' from rehab providers for giving tips on patients and referrals. Guardians are over-sold on the value, and likely outcome, of treatments, [the subcommittee] staff was told."

Some of these marketing techniques clearly involve outright conflict of interest and corruption of the judgment of professionals who have taken oaths to place the patient's welfare above opportunities for personal gain. Others, while not technically violating ethical standards, constitute extravagant expenditures on matters having nothing to do with patient care. Even many reputable acute-care hospitals, nursing homes, and for-profit rehabilitation companies with scientifically sound programs often engage in lavish marketing campaigns.

One for-profit brain-damage rehabilitation facility flew my research assistant to their facility for a visit and provided his meals and lodging. He was struck by the sixty-five-acre campus and its idyllic setting, the indoor and outdoor pools, and the rustic but tasteful architecture and decor. He was also impressed by the program, designed for sixty-eight "clients" at four different levels of recovery. He noted that the client to staff ratio was one-to-one for the most disabled patients, four-to-one for others, and that staff members were extremely well paid. At $539 per day, the average stay (six to nine months) cost $97,000 to $146,000. Still, he concluded, "after my visit, I would highly recommend this facility to those with the ability to pay and the appropriate need."

But other for-profit programs may do as much or more for patients and charge half the price, depending on the level of care that the patients require. True, accommodations may tend toward the spartan. Staff may be dedicated, but some may lack professional training. It is essential that the individual needs of patients be regularly evaluated by competent professionals and, ideally, coordinated by trained case managers. Some facilities charge patients on a sliding scale based on their ability to pay. Those who suffer from severe behavioral disturbances or are involved in intensive physical and vocational therapy pay more; those in the outpatient program pay less. The costs may range between three to twelve thousand a month, thus permitting longer periods of rehabilitation for less money.

Given rehabilitation programs of roughly equal quality, a victim of traumatic brain injury probably wouldn't notice much difference between facilities. But the patient's family might find the trappings at the upscale facility reassuring, and in almost every case, it is the family who makes the decision. If a facility presents an appearance and ambience somewhere between an elite summer camp and a rustic resort, it sends out the not-so-subtle message that the parents, spouse, or guardian have arranged the best rehabilitation that money can buy. In our culture we often make the mistake of confusing the most expensive with the best; we assume that the more we spend, the more we get. Slick promotional materials can make families feel guilty if they don't opt for expensive care, yet, given limited insurance settlements and personal financial resources, families might better serve their most vulnerable members by choosing facilities where the programs offer appropriate, individualized rehabilitation and the lower prices allow longer stays.

Many for-profit brain-trauma facilities do a good or even excellent job of providing essential services. Some also content themselves with a reasonable profit. The problem, as the Wyden subcommittee emphasized, is that this industry grew so rapidly and, in most states, without regulation. During the late 1980s, profits expanded 40 to 50 percent annually. Under these conditions, economic exploitation was bound to occur.

How did it happen in the late 1980s that large, private, for-profit medical businesses got away with systematic profiteering, fraud, and even patient abuse? Several factors combined to make it possible. First, there was a genuine lack of desperately needed services. Acute trauma care had improved dramatically over the preceding decade, which meant that thousands of patients who would formerly have died in fact survived. But our ability to rehabilitate them hadn't kept pace with our ability to save them. Because it isn't impeded by red tape or dependent on the generosity of individuals and foundations, the marketplace can respond much more quickly than government or charities can. If facilities and programs are needed and mechanisms are in place for providers to be paid, investors will rush to ante up the capital. Private enterprise responds rapidly to meet public demand for hospitals and nursing homes, just as it does to meet demand for restaurants, houses, and office buildings.

The key ingredient is huge amounts of cash in the hands of potential consumers. A large percentage of prospective patients have insurance—through automobile policies, workers' compensation, or employee health benefits—that covers the accidents that cause most traumatic brain injuries. During the 1980s, insurance companies paid claims to private facilities, and no one was responsible for oversight or regulation of the quality or even the legitimacy of the care these facilities provided.

In the post-acute-care phase, when victims of traumatic brain injury are focused on their need to overcome their physical, cognitive, and emotional problems, they are emotionally at their most vulnerable point. This is when they and their families make the easiest marks for the unscrupulous. Individuals who have survived severe brain injury face enormous challenges to recovery. They often suffer such movement disorders as spasticity, rigidity, tremors, tics, random jerks and restless shuffling, and distortions of posture and facial expression. Some patients are partially paralyzed. Others experience muscular weakness, difficulty maintaining balance, and mobility impairments. Neurological problems, such as epilepsy, hydrocephalus, and vascular complications, may arise after the person has left the hospital. Speech and other communication disorders can cause anything from mild to extreme loss of powers of expression and reception. Disorders of learning and memory, complex information processing, and perception are common consequences of brain trauma. So are personality disturbances like hallucinations, anxiety, depression, obsessional disorders, and inability to control sexual or aggressive impulses. Some patients are unable to carry out such simple activities of daily living as feeding and dressing themselves and maintaining personal hygiene.

Any of these disabilities alone or in combination interferes with an individual's ability to function in interpersonal settings. Even the most dedicated and supportive family members often lose patience when helping a child, spouse, or sibling with such problems. At the time that Robertson, Colman, and Stephens drafted their investment white paper, only 14 percent of the potential demand for inpatient brain-trauma rehabilitation services was being met. Many families who couldn't cope with brain-injured members were desperate to find some alternative to keeping them at home or warehousing them in a nursing home designed for the elderly, an entirely different population; families without financial resources would remain limited to those two options. But half of all traumatic brain injuries result from motor vehicle accidents, often accidents in which one driver or the other has insurance. Many of the falls that cause another one-fifth of brain traumas occur on the job; workers' compensation picks up the tab for rehabilitation, rightly figuring that doing so is usually less expensive than supporting the victim over a lifetime of disability. In the mid-1980s, plenty of brain-trauma victims weren't getting appropriate rehabilitation—not because they couldn't pay, but because so few facilities provided the lengthy rehabilitation and reeducation necessary for them to regain function.

Robertson, Colman, and Stephens drafted its bullish memo on traumatic brain injury during the height of the Reagan era, when the for-profit private sector was encouraged to step in and fill the needs traditionally met by government and by religious charities. And the private sector responded so quickly and enthusiastically that the number of brain-injury rehabilitation units covered by Medicare grew from about 350 in 1984 to about 825 in 1991.

These facilities—with their new buildings, attractive grounds, latest technologies and equipment, and enthusiastic marketing—fill an urgent need and provide hope and opportunities for patients and families. Undoubtedly, many patients do benefit from the full range of medical, psychological, and rehabilitative services offered. But if a rehabilitation facility promises *restoration* of function, patients and families may naively accept its unrealistic assurances. Euphoria and high expectations can turn to distress and disappointment when progress is slow or when it stops altogether, and the costs are enormous.

Some facilities promise services they never deliver, or they give patients fewer hours of these services than the marketing staff led the family to expect. Other rehabilitation centers deliver services that are inappropriate for the brain-trauma victim's present level of recovery. Compounding all this is the fact that because the field is so new and so few rigorous scientific studies have been completed, no one is quite sure which treatment techniques work and on whom.

Most brain-trauma victims who need rehabilitation aren't competent to assess the quality of care, let alone compare the value offered at one facility relative to another. Stressed and frustrated families are easy marks for upbeat and aggressive marketing, especially if they've already tried unsuccessfully to help their brain-damaged family member at home. The professionals who work in the facilities may be competent, well trained, and well intentioned, but they may overlook questionable and even unethical marketing practices because they find the work meaningful and the pay much better than they could earn in the public sector. The non-professional business staff may quiet their own misgivings by telling themselves that their company provides essential, high-quality services for a good cause and that aggressive marketing is essential to survival in a competitive marketplace. Pressured to maximize profits, they may decide to cut corners on less-visible functions, such as running thorough background checks on employees or providing adequate supervision for the night staff.

As a society, we need to permit the rehabilitation industry to generate reasonable profits, because the profit motive is still the best incentive we have, under our present system, for seeing that our most vulnerable citizens receive the services they need as quickly as possible. But we also need to regulate the industry closely to protect brain-trauma victims and their families from exploitation and to see that our collective resources are used prudently and effectively.

Using false promises, misleading advertising, and insurance

fraud to rake in huge profits is obviously illegal and immoral, and it victimizes all of us. The truth that none of us can afford to ignore is that the epidemic of traumatic brain injury costs enough, even without inflated profits, and that every dollar squandered could have been used to help another victim recover his or her fullest potential. The Wyden subcommittee found that the price of treating the eighty thousand to ninety thousand new victims of traumatic brain injury a year, plus all the previous years' survivors, is staggering. With young men from fifteen to twenty-four, the population group that is most likely to be injured, the annual bill now runs between $100,000 and $350,000 per patient. The lifelong cost for a single patient with severe disabilities comes to $4.6 million — enough money to send fifty undergraduates through Harvard.

In most states, residential facilities specializing in rehabilitation don't fall under normal licensing requirements for hospitals or nursing homes. Nor are there state or national standards for the treatment of the brain-injured. Rehabilitation of brain-trauma patients is interdisciplinary and complex, and it takes an average of five to ten years. Rivalries within the profession compound uncertainty about which treatments work. Although a peer-review accreditation program exists, most states don't require facilities to pass it. In theory, private insurance companies and Medicaid have control over the quality of care and the honesty and accuracy of billing, but oversight has been inadequate.

"If you look for a program affiliated with a not-for-profit hospital that has a community-based board, you'll find very few examples of the kind of greed that has afflicted some publicly traded companies," William Reynolds, director of the Bureau of Standards Development of the New York State Department of Health, advised in a recent interview. "You may have some people who are not as competent as you'd like them to be, but you don't have the pressure for them to cut corners and turn a short-term profit."

The brain-trauma rehabilitation industry relies on our culture's belief that every form of suffering has a quick fix, that some short-term solution can repair shattered brains and shattered lives. The tough truth is that no such magic bullet exists, and it never will. Even if sometime in the near or distant future biomedical research discovers a way to repair or regenerate damaged brain tissue, victims of severe head injuries will still need to relearn how to interpret visual data, how to read a bus schedule, even how and when to appropriately express sexual interest. Such reeducation may well require years.

No matter how reassuring and aesthetically pleasing the surroundings, no matter how good the food and how caring and competent the staff, an expensive resort masquerading as a rehabilitation center cannot offer a victim of traumatic brain injury a well-planned continuity of care in a two-month stay. Fortunately, there are many facilities that truly are trying to do their best for the vulnerable people they are pledged to help. These could do an even better job if they resisted the temptation to indulge in slick marketing and focused on ways to provide, within the constraints of average insurance coverage, the length of rehabilitation that their patients require.

Meanwhile, as a society, we need to focus our attention and resources on helping the brain-injured meet the long-term challenges of regaining function bit by bit, of maximizing potential, and of learning to live with disability as productively and as fully as possible.

Following the congressional subcommittee report, Congressman Wyden and Senators John D. Rockefeller IV and David Durenberger introduced the Brain Injury Rehabilitation Quality Act of 1992. The purpose of this legislation, in Congressman Wyden's words, was "to protect consumers against a rising tide of waste, fraud and abuse in this rapidly expanding field of health care."

Wyden listed a number of practices that rehabilitation centers were engaging in, including "denial of purchased services, overbilling, physically abusive treatment of patients, and the widespread use of questionable, ineffective or inappropriate treatments." The Brain Injury Rehabilitation Quality Act would have curbed many of these unethical and even illegal practices by instituting a case management system and creating a patient bill of rights. Yet despite clear evidence of problems within many of the rehabilitation centers and despite support from congressmen in both the House and Senate, the bill did not get passed, leaving vulnerable patients and their families unprotected by federal laws. Let us hope that these issues are revisited by Congress or state legislatures. Perhaps the passage of the 1996 Traumatic Brain Injury Act will help to renew interest in the public scrutiny of private practices.

A Better Use of Resources

You may recognize the following story: a beautiful young woman of royal birth falls into a persistent vegetative state and remains in it for many years—easily long enough for it to qualify as a permanent vegetative state. But as it turns out, her living in limbo is not permanent. Indeed, the young woman regains consciousness after a young man (a fellow royal) comes to pay his respects; when he touches her hand and kisses her lips, she opens her eyes and rises from her bed. Following a lightning-fast recovery, she is completely normal in every way, with absolutely no loss of function. She and the young man ultimately marry.

Unfortunately, such happy endings are mostly found where this one is—in a fairy tale. Beyond the story *Sleeping Beauty* and its modern movie equivalents, however, patients who regain consciousness after six months or a year in a persistent vegetative state don't blink a few times, ask in a clear voice, "Where am I? What happened?" and then smile wanly at their dedicated doctors and relieved loved ones. Instead, they emerge in tiny steps—eyes focused briefly on a person one day, an index finger raised on command weeks later. Their recovery goes only so far and then stops. But here the clinical uncertainty that attends all serious head injuries clouds the prognosis. The recovery process is so individual and subject to so many factors that neither neuroscientists nor rehabilitation therapists can predict its limits. Almost always, such patients are left with severe mental and physical disabilities.

Many times, the family of a PVS patient greets this tragic prognosis with denial. They disregard what doctors and nurses try to tell them and welcome the words of hopeful, upbeat friends, which help them feel better, regardless of the truth. But that sort of cheerfulness sets up the family for false hopes. In these circumstances, it's only human to hope for miracles, but they rarely happen. Such slim hopes may have a beneficial effect when they emotionally cushion the family who is adjusting to a head injury victim's plight. It may even be easier for the family to hold out for a miracle if the patient remains vegetative; if the injured regains consciousness, then the family is forced to confront his or her severe disabilities.

In 1994, I was called as a bioethicist to consult with defendants in a lawsuit brought by the family of Thon Nguyen (not his real name), a Vietnamese immigrant in his thirties who had been employed by a major construction firm in Houston. In May 1992, while he was working on a project at a petroleum refinery, he rode his bicycle into the back of a truck owned by the oil company. His head hit a protruding piece of metal with such force that it severely damaged most of the right side of his brain. Remarkably, Nguyen survived, but he was devastated. His only consistent response was reflexive withdrawal from painful stimuli. His accident also left him with a long list of medical problems ranging from respiratory infections to chronic diarrhea.

Because Nguyen was on the job at the time of his injury, workers' compensation paid his medical bills, but his family sued the oil company for pain and suffering and for a settlement to cover the cost of rehabilitation. At issue was whether he experienced or would ever be able to experience pain and suffering, or anything else. Another matter for debate was whether he could derive any sort of benefit from any kind of rehabilitation. Doctors who had examined the patient asserted that he was in a persistent vegetative state, completely unaware of his environment, and that he had shown no improvement in two years. He hadn't demonstrated an ability to understand simple commands in either English or Vietnamese. His only responses were reflexive. (A reflexive response to pressure didn't mean that he consciously *felt* the pain.) For these reasons, I was quite certain that Nguyen did not feel pain, would not do so in the future, and could not be helped by rehabilitation, but the family was prepared to field its own experts to argue otherwise.

It took the Houston hospital four and a half months to stabilize Nguyen enough for him to survive being transferred to Long Beach Memorial Medical Center near Los Angeles, where he could be close to his nearest family—his sister and her husband. After Nguyen had a stint in the intensive care unit, where he was treated again for respiratory problems and diarrhea, his doctors moved him to the subacute unit of a state-of-the-art rehabilitation facility near Los Angeles. This unit specialized in staving off medical complications while giving severely brain-injured patients the sensory stimulation that research shows might improve their cognitive functioning enough for them to take on more ambitious rehabilitation. Because it involved so much one-on-one work with a variety of professionals trained in sophisticated therapies, the program cost around fifteen hundred dollars a day. Nguyen's sister and brother-in-law demanded that he be kept there indefinitely at the oil company's expense. The company wanted to send him to a nursing home offering no rehabilitation but specializing in severe brain and nervous system disorders; its daily fee per patient was five hundred dollars.

By any neurological standard, Nguyen wasn't eligible for rehabilitation because he didn't have the capacity to benefit from it. Yet his sister, who visited him daily for months, claimed that he recognized her, even that he had talked to her. She and her husband consistently refused to sign "do not resuscitate" orders on his behalf and insisted that Nguyen would want everything possible done to preserve his life.

I was convinced that the sister was sincere, that she genuinely believed that her brother communicated with her. I was also quite certain that she was wrong. I'd seen many families of permanently vegetative patients pin similar false hopes on unconscious responses. Muscles contract and spasm on their own. In the imaginations of those denying the loss of loved ones, exhalations and coughs can become attempts to speak. The grasping reflex, which causes the hand of a newborn to curl around whatever touches the palm, exhibits itself in adults *only* when they have severe brain damage; yet it's comforting to interpret this very negative symptom as a positive responsive squeeze.

Several matters complicated the sister's reaction. Apparently, Nguyen had saved her life back in Vietnam, so she felt a strong obligation to repay the debt. If she thought she had abandoned him, the burden of guilt might be unbearable. Her concern for her brother also extended beyond this life. Although he had converted to Roman Catholicism, the rest of the family had remained Buddhist. Nguyen's sister feared that he would be reincarnated as a cockroach if he died without repenting of his womanizing and other misdeeds. But a Vietnamese Catholic priest familiar with Buddhist traditions said that he doubted such concerns applied to someone so severely brain-damaged. In the priest's opinion, continued treatment merely averted natural death.

A less noble complication also entered the picture. If Nguyen died, the lawsuit against the oil company would die with him. His family would get nothing. As long as he lived, the family had a shot at a lump-sum settlement for rehabilitation and at a big pain-and-suffering settlement, both a certain amount for their own distress and, if they could establish that Nguyen was conscious at least some of the time, a much larger amount for his. The bad outcome made for a good lawsuit.

Meanwhile, highly trained doctors, nurses, and therapists were giving state-of-the-art care to a man who couldn't possibly benefit from it, and other victims who might improve with appropriate rehabilitation were languishing in nursing homes—simply because their accidents hadn't happened at work or under conditions where the party at fault was well insured. In other words, these victims had been doubly unlucky.

That was certainly the case with Donny Michaels (not his real name), a patient whom I encountered as a result of a neurosurgeon's consultation request. Michaels could look at your face and in five minutes create a charcoal sketch that captured your features but exaggerated them in a way that revealed your personality. His caricatures were sometimes humorous, never mean, often uncanny. His evocative beach scenes and intricate abstract watercolors showed similar promise. People in the Gulf Coast resort town where he worked making quick portraits of tourists agreed that he had the talent and social skills to be a great deal more than a street artist—if only he weren't so fond of beer.

Making friends came easily to Michaels. His warmth, humor, and artistic perceptiveness charmed everyone from just-introduced acquaintances to his family. But his drinking and his constant requests for money strained his relationships. So did his periodic eruptions of paranoia.

Michaels lived for his art, allowing nothing to distract him from his work—except alcohol. In 1990, when he was thirty-one, Michaels's family confronted him about his drinking, but he insisted that he wouldn't—couldn't—give it up. A year later, Michaels attempted to kill himself by slitting his throat. Like many suicide attempts, this one was marked by ambivalence. Michaels had made sure that a friend knew where he was and what he planned to do, and he was rescued. Even after several weeks spent treating him in a psychiatric hospital, his psychotherapists couldn't decide whether his suicidal depression and other emotional problems represented an alcohol-induced disorder or a long-standing mental illness. The psychiatrist told Michaels's sister that Michaels would have to be sober for six months before a reliable assessment could be made. But in six months, Michaels was out of the hospital and back on the road, resuming his life as a nomadic artist.

Although in 1993 he sent his family a note warning them that someday he'd kill himself, the police officer who investigated his accident the next year said he had no reason to believe that it was another suicide attempt. On the night of Michaels's car wreck, Michaels had been engaged in what he called "maintenance beer drinking." Besides, it was four o'clock in the morning when he headed his 1986 Dodge toward the beach. As he approached the intersection, he may have dozed off momentarily. The impact of his car smashing into the utility pole threw Michaels's brain against its bony casing with such force that a large blood clot formed inside the back of his skull, putting increasing and potentially lethal pressure against the soft tissue.

Because a major medical center was only a few miles away, Michaels reached the emergency room less than an hour after his wreck, but even before the CT scan was performed, it was obvious that he'd suffered serious brain damage. Deeply unconscious, he responded only to pain, and then by extending his arms and legs rigidly rather than withdrawing from the pressure. The neurosurgeon didn't expect Michaels to survive surgery for the blood clot and the dislocated jaw and other injuries that he'd suffered in the crash. But the neurosurgeon was wrong. Despite the toll taken by twenty years of heavy drinking, Michaels's thirty-five-year-old body endured the trauma of the accident and the stress of the operation. He emerged physically alive but suspended in a persistent vegetative state.

For nearly two months, Michaels remained imprisoned in that limbo, unresponsive to commands, unaware of his environment, and unable to communicate. Then, to the surprise of the medical and nursing staff, he began to show signs of intermittent awareness—minimal but unmistakable evidence of visual and verbal interaction and the ability to follow simple commands. When his two older sisters and his mother came from out of state to visit, he recognized them. He even uttered a few words and sentences. Again, he'd defied his doctor's predictions.

Although Michaels has emerged from his persistent vegetative state, as I write his future is uncertain. He can move his arms and hands well enough to grasp and throw a soft Frisbee. With his left hand, he can even hold a pen and make marks on paper, but he has little if any control over his lower body. He seems to understand much of what people say to him, but his own speech is halting and difficult to understand, and the effort of maintaining consciousness quickly exhausts him. He may continue to recover brain function, but he may not. A stroke, a seizure, or a cardiac arrest could reverse the unexpected progress that he has made. For the severely brain-injured, the course of recovery is always unpredictable.

With a few years of appropriate rehabilitation, Michaels might recover enough to be able to again support himself as a sidewalk artist. He might be confined to a wheelchair but be able to live independently. But the services that he needs to improve cost money. Michaels is uninsured, and his family doesn't have the resources to help him. Like thousands of other indigent victims of traumatic brain injury, he will probably be discharged from the hospital to a nursing home, where Medicaid will pay for his custodial care but not his rehabilitation. This would be a tragedy, since it would leave him severely disabled but with just enough awareness of his situation to suffer loss, regret, frustration, and loneliness. It may also be a false economy, since two or three years invested in helping Michaels recover as much of his abilities as possible might save the taxpayers thirty or forty years of keeping him alive but totally dependent.

We spare no expense rescuing the seriously brain-injured but uninsured from untimely death, yet we seem unwilling to spend much, if anything, to prepare them for independent life. Once the trauma and acute-care teams have done their jobs and the patient is medically stable, further progress depends on the money available. In Nguyen's case, ample funds were there; in Michaels's, they weren't. A mason hit by a falling brick while working for a negligent but well-insured construction company will get state-of-the-art rehabilitation, often whether he seems to benefit from it or not. An uninsured man suffering the same injury while building a wall in his backyard will languish and decline in a nursing home, even if, like Michaels, he seems to be a good candidate for rehabilitation.

As members of a technologically advanced, relatively affluent society, we share a responsibility to see that all patients who are brain-injured but not persistently unconscious receive care that allows them to function at the highest level that they can achieve. Meanwhile, however, we are in the midst of a cost crisis: by the year 2000, rapidly inflating medical costs are expected to exceed $5,500 for every man, woman, and child in the country—a total of $1.5 trillion, or about 15 percent of the nation's gross domestic product. As the authors of *The New Medical Marketplace* have observed, in 1990 the United States spent nearly three times what Great Britain did on health care, yet average life expectancy and most other health indicators were about the same in the two countries. One reason we have not seen more positive results from our substantially greater outlays is that too often we put massive amounts of our limited resources into cases where it cannot possibly affect the outcome, as in the care of Thon Nguyen, instead of into cases where it might have a chance of getting individuals out of nursing homes and leading independent (or semi-independent) lives, as might be possible with Donny Michaels.

Of course, misallocating scarce resources among those with brain injuries is merely another illustration of how our current health care system, which is driven by misplaced financial incentives, frequently puts its money in the wrong places. Medicare, for instance, which represents nearly everyone of retirement age, spends enormous piles of cash on health care provided during the final six months of life. In any given case, most of the health care professionals involved (but not always the patient and his or her family) often know that there is virtually no hope of prolonging life beyond a few months—and sometimes know that aggressive treatment itself may diminish the quality of whatever life remains. In a number of such instances, informed patients might choose to see Medicare spend a smaller amount of money for palliative and lesser-skilled (or even unskilled) nursing care at home, thus allowing the terminally ill to die in familiar surroundings rather in the impersonal and expensive sterility of, say, a hospital's intensive care unit. But as things are now, they cannot make such choices, either because they aren't adequately informed about their options or because they can't afford this arguably more humane and cheaper alternative, which is not sufficiently covered by Medicare. As we lavish what is ultimately futile care on publicly or privately insured or well-off individuals with no hope of recovery, however, regular preventive medical treatment for the poor and uninsured, including poor children, is increasingly curtailed or unavailable. The upshot is that when the poor get sick, they wait until they are very sick and then visit public hospital emergency rooms—which costs society far more than catching the problems before they become medical emergencies.

While this discussion may seem to be ranging far afield from traumatic brain injury, the fact is that in cases of brain trauma (among many others), we can decide to take money currently spent on cases that are hopeless and redirect it to cases that may benefit from medical science. By actually doing so, we could not only save lives but salvage them as well. And we could accomplish this worthy goal with no more resources than we are spending today. But to really do it will require all of us—voters, policy makers, and politicians alike—to come to a meeting of the minds about how to reform our health care system and to make hard but rational choices about what treatments make sense and for whom.

When we fail to make necessary choices, we are in fact electing to continue in the same untenable patterns that we fall into at present, so it's important to focus on the human consequences of such inaction.

When we give brain-injury victims the care they need to save their lives but withhold the care they need to reach their potential, we compound the initial tragedy. Consider the case of Bobby Waldorf (not his real name). He was forty-five when his doctor told him that he had terminal cancer. Plummeted into a suicidal depression by the diagnosis, he shot himself in the head. His self-inflicted damage was extensive but not immediately fatal. A Life Flight helicopter rushed Waldorf to a hospital with a sophisticated trauma center, where he received excellent care soon enough after his injury to save him—at least for the time being.

His neurosurgeon reported that Waldorf had literally blown his brains out. Because the bullet left unprotected tissue exposed, the doctor predicted that Waldorf would die of an unavoidable and unstoppable brain infection. But after four months in the hospital, he was still alive. Although he'd survived, Waldorf had serious complications. He was paralyzed from the neck down, and his mental condition was severely compromised. He could engage in simple conversations but lacked the ability to function at a higher level of cognitive complexity. Ironically, the cancer that he had believed to be terminal was cured unexpectedly by radiotherapy. His suicide attempt had left him severely and permanently disabled, but he wasn't dying.

Because Waldorf was totally dependent, his wife, who had been appointed his legal guardian shortly after he shot himself, placed him in a nursing home not far from where she lived. After several years in the home, he developed ulcers on his legs, and they became infected. Bed sores like these are usually excruciating, but because Waldorf's brain damage had severed the nerves to his lower body, he felt no pain. Even so, his bed sores needed to be treated, and unbeknownst to his wife, the nursing home sent him to an acute-care hospital at the University of Texas Medical Branch at Galveston, which accepts patients without regard to ability to pay. When Waldorf's wife discovered that he had been transferred without her approval, she was furious. When the hospital asked her to consent on his behalf to antibiotic medication for the sores, she refused. She argued that since he was experiencing no pain, the sores did not need treatment, even though she knew that Waldorf might die from the infection. She said, "God should be allowed to finish what Bobby started."

The attending physician consulted me for advice. She believed that she had a duty as a doctor to treat a life-threatening condition, but she was hesitant to treat Waldorf over the objections of his legal guardian—at least not without some assurance that the law permitted her to do so. After consulting with the legal counsel for the hospital, I advised the physician that we should talk to Waldorf first to determine his preferences. Waldorf seemed to comprehend that his infected bed sores needed treatment; at least he was willing to undergo the recommended course of antibiotics even if he didn't fully understand the details of what was being proposed. Under these circumstances, the physician felt that she was obligated to try to save her patient's life, and I agreed.

Although Waldorf's wife was unhappy about the situation, she didn't persist in her protests. She did warn the hospital that she wouldn't be able to visit her husband or attend to his personal needs as she had when he was in a nearby nursing home. She lived more than seventy-five miles from Galveston and needed to work to support herself. Waldorf's treatment succeeded in curing his bed sores, but the nursing home that had transferred him to our hospital refused to readmit him. The nearest facility where he could be placed was even farther from his wife than we were. She stopped visiting him completely. Since Waldorf had no other close family, he was cut off from his only important personal relationship. A few months later, Bobby Waldorf died alone at the distant nursing home.

In a world of more abundant resources or more rational policies, it would be easier to find a more acceptable solution to Waldorf's problem. If he or his wife had had more money or better health insurance, he might have been treated at a hospital closer to his home. If whoever first told his wife that his bed sores required medical treatment had discussed the ramifications clearly, she might have been able to negotiate with the nearby nursing home to readmit him after he left the hospital. If his rights had been protected better from the outset, that nursing home might have been required to readmit him.

When individuals so severely disabled that they can't care for their own needs or assert their rights are cut off from their families and friends and lack other advocates, they face a fate similar to

Waldorf's. Many people knew that Waldorf's needs weren't being met, but his welfare was subordinated to the pressures of a system of care that could save his life but not preserve its quality.

We must be fair to patients devastated by traumatic brain injury, but we must also be realistic. We should certainly direct resources toward improving assessment tools so that we can evaluate patients better and earlier, even as we recognize that determining an individual's potential for progress may never be an exact science.

Because severely brain-injured patients may survive for long periods in an unconscious state, we need to establish policies that provide the opportunity for recovery, even to the limited level possible for someone like Bobby Waldorf, but don't encourage futile efforts for hopeless cases like Thon Nguyen's. Such cases will always be surrounded by ambiguity, and deciding what level of care is appropriate in each instance will never be easy. But our current failure to confront this challenge is unacceptable. Our ambivalence compounds tragedy with inequity. The cost of maintaining a patient without medical complications in the limbo of permanent unconsciousness is about $150,000 per year. The same time spent in a good inpatient rehabilitation program runs around $300,000 annually. For what it costs to preserve the mere organic existence of two permanently vegetative brain-damaged individuals, we could help a devastated patient with a better prognosis achieve his or her highest potential, perhaps even trade a life of total dependency for one of self-reliance and contribution.

Policies and Priorities

In the United States we would do well to make combating traumatic brain injury a national priority. With the exceptions of heart disease, cancer, and stroke, traumatic brain injury is the greatest public health crisis that we face today. Compared to AIDS, brain injuries account for 60 percent more deaths and afflicts an even younger population, killing and disabling more children and young adults than any other cause. From the beginning of 1945 to the end of 1994, brain trauma caused more than 2.5 million fatalities and 25 million injuries in the United States. Clearly, we must take action against this epidemic. In recent years, we've made a start, but we must move forward more quickly and deliberately than we have in the past. Fortunately, the measures that I discuss in this chapter and the next are concrete and practical. Some of them will cost money, but many involve spending no more than we spend now.

The first step that we as a society must take to combat traumatic brain injury is to focus attention on it as a pressing menace to the health and well-being of us all. Although neuroscientists, rehabilitation professionals, and a few journalists are taking more notice of brain trauma, the public profile of this epidemic remains far too low.

Every year, about 800,000 Americans die from heart and cardiovascular disease, about 500,000 from cancer, and about 150,000 from strokes. During that same period, at least 60,000 Americans die from brain trauma (a conservative estimate; others suggest 75,000 to 100,000), about the same number who die from Alzheimer's disease; another 70,000 to 90,000 survive but face a lifetime of severe disability. Diabetes and its complications (including disorders related to elevated blood sugar but included in overall cardiovascular statistics) do kill more people—160,000 Americans a year—but diabetes isn't as devastating a disabler. Unfortunately, there is no equivalent to insulin in helping brain-trauma victims to function.

Brain trauma robs us of $7.6 billion annually: $2.9 billion are in direct costs, including treatment, rehabilitation, and care; $4.7 billion arise from indirect costs, including lost wages, taxes, and productivity. And the emotional price paid by the victims and their families, friends, and co-workers makes brain trauma one of the most tragic of all human afflictions. We can't afford to keep ignoring it.

Even if we or members of our families never suffer severe brain trauma, we all pay the bill. Young men between the ages of fifteen and twenty-four, those at highest risk for head injuries, are also those least likely to have insurance. As many as 40 million Americans have no health insurance, and in many of our most populous states, including New York and California, between 15 and 25 percent of all drivers are uninsured as well. Although all of us are vulnerable, a study conducted in San Diego in 1986 found that people with household incomes under $15,000 were half again as likely to suffer serious brain injuries as people making more. Poverty and the stresses that it imposes seem to put people at risk for falls, violence, and traffic accidents. When the poor and uninsured have brain injuries, we end up sharing their medical bills through state and federal taxes.

Yet traumatic brain injury seldom comes to mind when we list major public health problems. We all know about cancer and cardiovascular disease. Not only are they so common that almost everyone has known someone who has suffered from them; these afflictions usually hit in middle and late life, striking many of their victims at the height of their prosperity and power, when they have the means to focus public attention on whatever threatens them.

Like AIDS, traumatic brain injury disproportionately hits the young and those in their prime. In 1995, AIDS took 35,607 American lives—a terrible toll, but only half the number who died that year from brain trauma. Yet, thanks to effective advocacy, we are far more aware of AIDS than we are of severe head injury. Billboards, public service announcements, television programs, and newspaper and magazine stories have informed the American public of the threat posed by AIDS and of ways to reduce their vulnerability to infection.

One reason for the failure to give traumatic brain injury the attention it deserves is that we seldom identify it as a single entity. Instead, we tend to look at the separate causes: car, truck, and motorcycle accidents; falls, violence, and sports injuries. We don't look at the unifying calamity that constitutes their most serious result. Paradoxically, as with statistics on cancer, heart disease, and stroke, the numbers of victims are large enough to surprise and even shock us, yet so large that we have trouble comprehending them. They become abstractions and are therefore easy to disregard. As recounted in the newspapers, the individual cases are dramatic; they move us to sympathy, but only with a single victim and his or her family at a time. As Joseph Stalin is said to have observed, "One man's death is a tragedy; a hundred thousand deaths is a statistic."

Statistics are general and abstract; case studies are singular and concrete. Neither capture the magnitude of the suffering of thousands of individuals and families; nor can they convey the successes and failures, triumphs and frustrations, and sheer number of hours of painstaking effort on the part of physicians, neuroscientists, and physical, behavioral, speech, and occupational therapists.

It is difficult for anyone to truly comprehend the searing impact of traumatic brain injury. Sometimes detailed narratives can come close to communicating its complexity, urgency, and propensity for causing human devastation—I think of A. R. Luria's compelling *The Man with a Shattered World,* a book about one of Luria's patients. But we must often resort to art, symbolic representation, or metaphor to approach full understanding of a brain-trauma victim's individual experience. And even that lived experience, as conveyed to us, is bound to be only partial, because by its very nature, traumatic brain injury steals the memories, thoughts, and fantasies that accompany the trauma and its aftermath.

Still, we work with what we have and use it for our specific purposes. Epidemiologists seek to get an accurate quantitative picture of the incidence and prevalence of a defined phenomenon. Journalists want to tell a gripping, relevant story. Advocacy groups strive to raise awareness and generate support for their cause. Policy makers must decide which social problems should be addressed with legislation, regulation, and funding and must determine the order in which they should be tackled.

In general, Americans have been slow to identify injury as a public health issue. Not until 1992 did the Centers for Disease Control and Prevention, responding to pressure from policy makers, establish the Center for Injury Prevention and Control. In 1989, Dorothy P. Rice, former director of the National Center for Health Statistics, and Ellen J. MacKenzie, assistant director of the Health Services Research and Development Center at Johns Hopkins University, reported to Congress that in 1985 injuries of all types cost the country $158 billion. They also found that vehicular accidents, the biggest cause of brain trauma, were also the single greatest cause of the most expensive injuries; car, truck, and motorcycle mishaps accounted for 9 percent of all injuries but for 31 percent of the resulting costs over a lifetime. Falls, the second largest cause of traumatic brain injury, came in second in injury-related expense, accounting for 24 percent of lifetime expenditures. Firearms, still another major brain-trauma culprit, placed third in cost. The brutal fact is that brain damage is not only devastating in itself; it is also devastatingly expensive to treat and to live with.

RESEARCH

Our reluctance to confront traumatic brain injury as a health crisis exhibits itself clearly in the disparity in research funding. Both the National Cancer Institute and the National Institute of Neurological Disorders and Stroke (NINDS) are part of the National Institutes of Health (NIH), the agency that acts as a conduit for the federal money invested in research. While each NIH institute does undertake some limited inquiries into the diseases or disabilities that it was founded to address, its primary function isn't to conduct its own research but to support studies conducted by others, primarily researchers at health sciences universities. Leaving aside the millions of dollars that drug companies put into product development and testing, the NIH controls an overwhelming proportion of the money invested in examining the mysteries of how the human body functions and what can be done to promote health and combat disease and disability. By comparison, even the highest-profile nonprofit foundations contribute only a small fraction. For example, in 1993 the American Cancer Society (whose primary mission is education) awarded less than $4 million in research grants; that same year, the National Cancer Institute spent over $2 billion—more than 425 times that amount.

With that kind of financial clout, the NIH sets the country's research priorities. As a public entity responsive to an elected Congress, it also roughly reflects how important our society considers each affliction. Each year, cancer kills seven to ten times the number of Americans killed by traumatic brain injury. We invest $2 billion annually in cancer research; by a strict proportional standard, we should be investing between $200 million and $285 million in research related to traumatic brain injury.

Instead, the NINDS spent a little over a tenth of that—just $29,235,000—researching head injury and related trauma in 1993 and roughly the same amount in 1994.

And that modest figure represents what the country is devoting to brain-trauma research during what is intended to be a concerted effort to expand basic and clinical knowledge of the body's most complex organ. In 1989, President George Bush signed Public Law 101–58 declaring the 1990s the Decade of the Brain and funneling additional funds to the NINDS. The institute asked for a total of $901 million to fund the first year of the Decade of the Brain. The institute's wish list covered fifteen areas of inquiry. In terms of amount of funding requested, the top three areas were cerebral palsy and other developmental disorders ($113.5 million), stroke and cerebrovascular disease ($91.2 million), and nerve and muscle disorders ($77.2 million). Traumatic brain injury came in tenth ($55.1 million), after epilepsy, multiple sclerosis, inherited disorders, and spinal cord injuries. And by the time the congressional budget paring was over, even this modest allocation had been slashed by almost half—despite the fact that traumatic brain injury kills and disables more Americans than do any of these disorders except stroke and cerebrovascular disease.

By the end of 1994, the National Institute of Neurological Disorders and Stroke had established three comprehensive brain-injury research centers and eight centers to test promising treatments. By the close of the decade, it hopes to have a network of fifteen clinical centers dedicated to traumatic brain injury and to spend $78.2 million per year on related research. But in order to reach that goal, it will have to overcome our reluctance to confront the reality of the brain-trauma epidemic, our denial of our own vulnerability to brain injury, and our resistance to spending public money on anything for which we can't see a potential personal benefit.

Before new knowledge gained from basic research can be used to help brain-trauma victims, the therapies that it makes possible must undergo rigorous clinical trials. Each such study typically costs about $5 million altogether; spread over five years, that amount funds about twenty grants. In cancer, some innovative treatments are in their third or fourth round of clinical trials. In traumatic brain injury, many promising treatments discussed in Chapter 3, such as hypothermia, haven't completed their first—not because of a lack of science but because of a lack of funding. Some of these would offer enormous benefits if they were proved to be safe and effective for a broad range of patients.

RETHINKING REHABILITATION

In focusing more attention on traumatic brain injury, we do need to increase our investment in basic and clinical research, at least bringing it into line with what we spend on investigating conditions that afflict far fewer people. But as we raise the level of funding, we also need to be careful not to merely perpetuate the crisis thinking that has hampered our ability to effectively confront brain injury. Biomedical research appeals to our infatuation with heroic solutions—rescue for an individual patient, cure for a disease. After all, Americans respond well to emergencies, a predisposition that partly explains our impressive advances in trauma care. Now neuroscience is extending further, probing ways to repair and replace damaged brain tissue. But this is still a medical approach based on a medical model. It seduces us into looking at a battered brain as we might look at a broken leg or a severed spine, mistakenly assuming that once the physical damage is healed, function can resume—that if only we could figure out how to repair the wound, we would solve the problem.

But the brain has more than a physical dimension. It has cognitive, emotional, social, aesthetic, and (one can argue) spiritual dimensions as well. Once a broken leg heals properly and completely, a brief exercise regimen usually restores complete function. Neurologists appear to be on the brink of being able to mend spinal breaks that previously resulted in paralysis; the physical therapy that follows may be longer and more involved, but it still will be straightforward.

Not so with traumatic brain injury. Regardless of future breakthroughs in the medical treatment of brain trauma, it now seems, recovery will remain complicated and uncertain. We mustn't delude ourselves into thinking that medical science will find every answer to this problem.

No amount invested in basic and clinical investigations will relieve us of our ongoing collective responsibility. Traumatic brain injury is not like smallpox or polio—it is not a blight that we can defeat once and for all with a concerted and sustained medical offensive. It will always be with us, either in its current state or as a reduced but looming threat. Confronting it effectively demands continuous effort and some fundamental changes, both in our individual attitudes and actions and in our culture as a whole.

We are already taking the first steps. Research is moving beyond medical treatment and into rehabilitation, where it is sorely needed. For too long, rehabilitation following brain trauma has been a matter of trial and error, with no sound basis for determining what worked and what didn't—or why. The National Institute of Neurological Disorders and Stroke is funding some programs in neuropsychology aimed at discovering exactly how brain trauma disrupts learning, thinking, and behavior and providing solid scientific underpinnings for the development of new rehabilitation methods. But for the most part, despite recent interest in brain-injury rehabilitation, there is scant scientific evidence for the claims that rehabilitation institutions make about their treatments. For instance, researchers tend to agree that, in order to reroute neural pathways around areas damaged by trauma, the healing brain needs stimulation. Thus a patient recently emerged from coma does best in a well-lighted room with people around and music playing. But whether music has some special effect beyond what a radio talk show might impart, and whether Vivaldi or the Rolling Stones might be a better choice, no one knows.

What studies have been conducted to test the efficacy of various rehabilitation methods haven't been nearly as rigorous as past trials of treatments for the acute stage of traumatic brain injury. One problem is that few rehabilitation institutions seem willing to submit their favorite therapies to the scrutiny of controlled trials. Furthermore, many of the publications about rehabilitation are sponsored by the rehabilitation institutions themselves; while the preliminary reports that the publications include may be interesting and even important, they can't be considered definitive because they haven't stood the test of unbiased examination and evaluation.

Another problem with rehabilitation research is that measuring the results is much more difficult and complex than measuring the results of acute intervention. Each brain injury is unique, each victim is unique, and each exists in a unique environment. At the initial rescue and acute stages, healing is a physical process; the underlying mechanisms are similar from one person to another and therefore relatively amenable to objective valuation. The factors involved in recovery after that point, however, are much harder to pin down. Although experience has taught experts that motivation, persistence, and family support are important to a brain-trauma victim's rehabilitation, ingredients like these don't easily lend themselves to quantification. But research is gradually moving onto this slippery terrain. The National Institute of Neurological Disorders and Stroke, for example, has funded a study comparing the recoveries of children whose traumatic brain injuries resulted from falls and other accidents with those of children whose brains were damaged by abuse.

The National Institute on Disability and Rehabilitation Research (NIDRR) appears to be well on its way to breakthroughs for the head-injured. Rather than being affiliated with the National Institutes of Health, NIDRR is part of the Department of Education, which gives it a perspective more appropriate to the difficult road faced by victims of traumatic brain injury and their families. It has designated two centers to conduct medical research into brain trauma. In addition, it has designated four model rehabilitation systems—the Santa Clara Valley Medical Center in San Jose, Wayne State University in Detroit, the Medical College of Virginia in Richmond, and The Institute for Rehabilitation and Research (TIRR) in Houston. Each of these has developed and is evaluating a comprehensive program for delivering services to victims of traumatic brain injury, from the moment of the trauma through reintegration into society.

The emphasis on education and the long term is important. "A head-trauma victim's actual physical impairment may not change after a year and a half, when neurological healing plateaus," explains

Don Lehmkuhl, a neurophysiologist and the director of the Re-habilitation Research and Training Center on Rehabilitation Inter-ventions Following Traumatic Brain Injury at TIRR. "But through education and by changing the environment, we can improve that person's ability to function in the community."

In February 1994, NIDRR awarded TIRR an additional five-year grant of $650,000 per year to develop the center that Dr. Lehm-kuhl runs and to find valid and reliable ways of measuring each patient's outcome. Until researchers have meaningful data that per-mit comparison, they won't be able to investigate how well various rehabilitation methods work. Most existing outcome measures at-tempt to reflect the patient's degree of impairment and disability, but TIRR is testing two scales for gauging the patient's ability to perform specific social roles: the Craig Handicap Assessment and Reporting Technique (CHART) and the Community Integration Questionnaire (CIQ). The CHART has five subscales: physical inde-pendence, mobility, occupation, social integration, and economic self-sufficiency. The CIQ has three: home integration, social integra-tion, and productivity. The mark of successful rehabilitation isn't whether the person with a brain injury has to use a wheelchair but how well that individual in a wheelchair can accomplish the tasks of daily living, perform in a job, and relate to others.

Devising new therapies and testing existing ones is important, but we must not forget that for therapies to be truly effective, they must be available to those who need them. Although critics may question the efficacy of some techniques and most regimens have yet to withstand the rigor of scientific testing, there are others, such as the exercises involved in speech therapy, that rehabilitation professionals have shown do work. The problem is that access to such services usually depends on insurance and other financial re-sources as well as on where the patient lives rather than on his or her potential for benefiting from them. Extending the frontiers of rehabilitation research is a worthy endeavor, but it is of limited use unless we apply what we learn to everyone who needs help and not just to those lucky enough to be able to pay for it.

Assuring that the brain-injured receive the rehabilitation they need—and only the rehabilitation they can benefit from—also entails seeing that providers of these services are properly trained and that the people in their care are neither neglected nor abused. The business of rehabilitation has mushroomed into a multi-billion-dollar industry free of regulation. To protect this vulnerable population, public agencies and private professional associations must establish standards for the training and competency of therapists and for the management of rehabilitation facilities.

HELP WITH LIVING

Beyond these moral and pragmatic challenges is one that is even tougher: no matter how much money and effort we put into it, no matter how fairly and rationally we distribute services, rehabilitation doesn't always work. The rhetoric of rehabilitation continues to focus on recovery and improvement, but for many thousands of brain-injury survivors, recovery has in fact plateaued and subsequent improvement, if any, will be very small. What do we do with this large population of chronically disabled individuals who are never going to get much better? Who will provide the support services they need to function at even the level of basic survival? At present, Medicaid and Medicare fund minimal services, doing better in some states than in others. The primary burden falls to the families, most of whom become overwhelmed by the costs and daily challenges.

Our society must come to terms with this issue. Just as our responsibility doesn't end when we've saved the life of a person with a serious brain injury, it doesn't end when we've given that individual appropriate rehabilitation. Although universal access to these services will maximize the percentage of brain-injured who regain independence and are able to support themselves, some won't be so lucky. Providing the most seriously disabled with appropriate housing, food, supervision, transportation, social and psychological counseling, medical care, and the other necessities of life is society's collective responsibility. Shifting this burden to the families only creates more victims and robs us of the other contributions that caretaking individuals would otherwise make. Besides, some people who suffer brain injuries don't have families, and others' families are unwilling or unable to take care of them. We should accept the burden, both because we have a moral obligation to help the needy and because traumatic brain injury could happen to any of us, causing us to require the same assistance ourselves.

Since many progressive programs for helping brain-injured individuals have come from the states, as a matter of policy the federal government should provide funding and broad guidelines but leave sufficient latitude for states to develop or institute innovative programs for providing and regulating services. In this way, the federal government could focus chiefly on funding research, collecting data on the causes and incidence of brain trauma, establishing rigorous standards for the rehabilitation industry, and educating Americans about brain trauma. States that have yet to put programs in place could select the strategies that have worked well elsewhere and modify these to make them appropriate to their populations. If the legislatures fail to act on this issue, the media and, one hopes, informed voters can add their voices to those of brain-trauma interest groups and make sure every representative understands that programs in place in other states are cost-effective ways of delivering essential services. It's up to all of us to transform the silent epidemic into one heard and responded to in the places where public policy is made.

Even after appropriate rehabilitation, many survivors of traumatic brain injury need public help in order to maintain their highest possible level of function. If they aren't capable of living by themselves, society should provide them with group housing or give their families financial assistance to defray the cost of their care and of necessary alterations to their homes, such as doorways that have to be widened or bathrooms altered to accommodate wheelchairs. Often, brain-injured individuals can live semi-independently in an appropriately modified environment if they are given regular help with chores and access to public transportation. They also may benefit from vocational training and job placement. Many recover normal levels of intelligence but have persistent problems with integrating knowledge; further encouraging employers to develop suitable positions—as the Americans with Disabilities Act does to some extent—may transform the brain-injured from lifelong dependents to contributing members of society.

Giving brain-trauma victims and their families the services from which they can benefit not only is the right thing for a civilized society to do; it also makes economic sense. Why, then, have we taken so long to get around to it, and why are we still dragging our feet?

CHANGING OUR ATTITUDES

Before we can take effective collective action against the epidemic of brain trauma, we must deal with our ambivalence and discomfort with brain injury and its victims. Severe brain trauma interferes with the very interpersonal and communication skills that human beings use to elicit understanding and caring from others. A person whose speech is halting and slurred evokes pity but not empathy. The sight of a previously normal adult reduced to the mental capacity of a young child and barely able to sit upright in a wheelchair is so horrible to contemplate that we tend to turn away. We feel impotent in the face of the tragedy and confused about what response would be appropriate. We also experience a desperate, albeit often unconscious, need to erect an emotional wall between us and the unfortunate individual, attempting to reassure ourselves that a similar fate couldn't befall us—although, of course, it could. We even tend to disregard fatigue, judgment lapses, short-term memory deficits, and other effects of minor brain injury in family members and co-workers. Loss of mental capacity in ourselves and changes in the personalities of those close to us are two of the most nightmarish situations imaginable. No wonder we recoil from the brain-injured.

As we do with AIDS, we often resort to blaming the victim, especially if the injury involved some element of voluntary risk taking. That twelve-year-old girl shouldn't have taken up horseback riding, or she should have worn a helmet. That seventeen-year-old boy shouldn't have been driving eighty miles an hour, especially without fastening his seat belt. And as for the parents who for the rest of their lives will be caring for a disabled daughter or son, they should never have bought the horse or handed over the keys to the car. That middle-aged woman should have called a cab instead of trying to drive home after three drinks. That elderly man shouldn't have been living in a house with stairs.

In September 1992, Jean Ann McLaughlin testified before the U.S. Senate in favor of Senator Ted Kennedy's traumatic brain injury bill, which finally became law in 1996. In a voice rendered halting by lingering speech defects, she gave a poignant description of living with the disabilities that plague hundreds of thousands of people with brain injuries. McLaughlin had suffered her catastrophe under circumstances well beyond her control; while operating her car at a normal speed, she had been hit head-on by a drunk driver. Yet, as she spoke, members of the audience fidgeted uncomfortably and averted their eyes. Another witness at the hearing, Clark Watts, a neurosurgeon and the director of the shock trauma center at the University of Maryland Medical Center, explained to reporter Laurie Jones that this was a typical reaction. "Everyone gets uncomfortable—they don't know where to look and they can't wait to get out of there," he said. "It's not like having an eloquent Hollywood wife who got infected with HIV through a transfusion address a national political convention. People don't squirm at that."

Such self-protective reactions may help us turn the tragedies of others into cautionary tales that encourage us to practice safer behavior, and they may give us the collective will to enact legislation and even change our culture in order to prevent traumatic brain injury. But they don't relieve us of our obligation to help those who are already its victims.

Despite the recent phenomenal expansion of rehabilitation facilities, only 5 percent of the victims of traumatic brain injury receive the rehabilitation services that they need to reach their maximum potential for recovery. Despite recent strides in brain research, severe traumatic brain injury remains a medical disaster, because recovery is usually lengthy, often incomplete, and always uncertain. Brain trauma is an economic crisis because care is expensive, rarely covered adequately by insurance, and uneven in its efficacy. Patients with substantial financial resources can obtain elaborate rehabilitation services, even if these do them little or no good, while patients of modest or straitened circumstances rarely receive enough rehabilitation, even if that care is likely to make the difference between a lifetime of expensive public dependency and one of self-support or at least relative self-sufficiency.

This makes no rational sense. It makes no medical sense. It makes no moral sense. On top of that, it is unfair. Unfortunately, it is all too typical of our nation's health care system.

One of the essential tenets of any civilized society is a commitment to assist and protect its neediest members. When a person suffers a serious head injury, that person needs our assistance and protection. Our moral sense tells us that acting together as a society, we must do whatever is reasonable to help. Our rational sense tells us that "help" in this sense entails doing what we believe offers the greatest promise for fulfilling that need in the long run. Because our resources are always finite and our collective obligation extends to so many individuals, we can—in fact we should—apply demanding standards of effectiveness and efficiency to the help we give; but we can't abandon the needy.

I have no delusions that our system can be made wholly rational and fair. But most people who stop to think about it believe that anyone in need of emergency life-saving care should get it. Emergency medical technicians don't check a trauma or heart-attack victim's wallet for proof of insurance before stabilizing that person and rushing him or her to the hospital. We agree that any human being in that predicament deserves a fair chance to survive and thrive. That is what we would want for ourselves under similar circumstances.

But when confronted with applying these precepts, we seem unable to go beyond the first step. We tell our rescue and trauma teams to spare no effort and expense in saving the victim's biological life. Then, once continued survival is likely, we disclaim further responsibility. We become distracted by irrelevant considerations, irrational fears, and lack of respect and concern for others. Because we don't like to face our own mean-spiritedness and vulnerability, because we don't want to admit our own bias and bigotry, we blame the victims of traumatic brain injury, devalue them as people, and argue that we don't have the resources to help them. We make decisions that make no sense, even from a purely economic point of view. We permit and support the system that I described in Chapter 8, the system that denies the severely brain-injured but alert street artist Donny Michaels the rehabilitation services that might enable him to become self-supporting, yet lavishes futile and costly treatment on Thon Nguyen, who is in a persistent vegetative state due to an accident that involved a well-insured oil company.

HOW WE CAN PAY FOR PROGRESS

A rational, coordinated, morally responsible approach to traumatic brain injury would benefit us all, indirectly if not directly. We need to inform ourselves and our families, friends, and co-workers. We must press our political representatives and other policy makers to give brain trauma the attention it deserves.

We must recognize that money spent wisely on stemming the brain-trauma epidemic is money well invested. Of course, we have to hold treatment, therapy, service, and research programs to high standards of appropriateness and cost-effectiveness, but this is not an area where we can afford to scrimp. Because in one way or another we all bear the cost of every victim's brain trauma, maintaining the current parsimonious level of funding is shortsighted in the extreme.

We neglected society's best interests when we allowed Congress to retreat from expanding Medicare to include insurance for catastrophic care for the elderly. That program would have covered treatment for traumatic brain injury, as well as other lengthy afflictions, in Americans sixty-five years of age and older. Although federal legislation for such coverage passed in 1988, it was revoked the following year after a coalition of interest groups, led by the American Association of Retired Persons, suddenly realized that the program would require each person eligible for Medicare to pay a surtax for catastrophic coverage, with the better-off segment paying proportionally more. The idea behind the legislation was popular—but only if no one had to pay for its fruition.

Catastrophic health insurance was a good idea. Its reversal was a prime example of both collective and individual shortsightedness. Instead of killing the legislation, Congress should have extended it to cover all Americans, not just Medicare recipients.

This progressive legislation was killed by a paradox: few people can afford catastrophic health care. Even three or four months of treatment for cancer or a serious heart defect can easily deplete substantial savings or exceed the lifetime-benefit limit of the standard insurance policy. Yet the chance of any one of us developing a brain tumor or needing a triple bypass is relatively low, and people are reluctant to support programs that are unlikely to benefit them personally. Persuading them to do so requires strong, committed leadership, and that's in short supply. Most contemporary politicians are more comfortable following polls and adjusting their votes accordingly than presenting strong arguments for meritorious programs that lack superficial appeal.

The debate about more sweeping health care reform and universal access that occupied the first two years of the Clinton administration swept aside separate discussion about catastrophic care. But now that this more ambitious agenda has been shelved, we should resurrect the earlier subject, this time directing more effort toward presenting the compelling arguments for universal catastrophic health insurance.

Precisely because it's unlikely that any given individual will suffer a long, expensive affliction, insurance premiums for catastrophic care policies can be set at affordable rates. Like any form of insurance, it's a gamble, but it can prevent a medical catastrophe from becoming an economic catastrophe or worse.

If every victim of traumatic brain injury had good catastrophic health coverage, every victim would be able to afford the rehabilitation necessary to reach his or her highest possible level of functioning. The chief barrier to access would be geographic. People living in big cities would have a range of programs near their homes, all competing to offer the most effective rehabilitation services. Victims in small towns and rural communities might have to seek care located hours away from their families. But at least everyone with severe brain trauma would be able to find help somewhere.

We could pay for universal catastrophic health care insurance by collecting the modest premiums along with federal income taxes, as we do with mandatory contributions to Social Security. After that, we would still need to figure out a way to fund research into promising medical and rehabilitation therapies. And we would need to do the same to cover the cost of statewide coordinating agencies to regulate, oversee, and support the rehabilitation industry and to direct the brain-injured and their families to the appropriate services. And beyond that, to be both just and rational, we would need to come up with the money to provide appropriate transportation, social and occupational services, and living arrangements for brain-injured individuals who, despite the best rehabilitative care, make only partial recoveries.

One fair strategy for generating the money to deal with these expenses is for federal and state governments to tax those activities that are the biggest contributors to brain trauma. Since vehicles are the number-one culprit, an extra dollar or two added to driver's license and registration fees and earmarked for brain-trauma rehabilitation would be appropriate. So would a few cents more per gallon at the gas pump. Licenses for drivers under twenty-five, who cause a disproportionate number of accidents, could carry an additional surcharge. Until we enact a universal, national catastrophic-care plan, states could cover the costs of more than half of these injuries by requiring motorists to carry automobile insurance policies that include acute, rehabilitative, and long-term care for traumatic brain injury. The states could also establish reserves to extend these benefits to people hurt by drivers who, despite the law, were uninsured. Because the likelihood is slight that any individual driver or passenger will suffer serious brain trauma in an accident, the additional premium shouldn't amount to more than 10 percent of the cost of a policy without this protection.

In 1991, Texas set up a trust fund for victims of brain and spinal cord injuries. Administered by the Texas Rehabilitation Commission, the money comes from a twenty-five-dollar surcharge on fines for driving under the influence and a five-dollar surcharge on other moving violations. Florida operates a similar fund, paying for it with 8.2 percent of all civil penalties collected by the county courts.

Because alcohol consumption increases the likelihood of both vehicular accidents and falls, the second most frequent cause of brain injuries, raising the tax on beer, wine, and liquor would be fair and appropriate; some of that money could also go to repairing the nontraumatic forms of brain damage caused by alcohol. Assaults rank third as a cause. Because assaults, including assaults with firearms, make up the third biggest cause of brain trauma, governments should impose fees on guns and ammunition and earmark the monies for treatment of brain trauma. Part of the price of every ticket sold to a boxing match should go toward correcting the devastation caused by this sport.

Think what our society could do with the proceeds from a 5 or 10 percent tax on all such risky activities. It would give our country billions of dollars a year to spend on not only prevention campaigns but also rehabilitation, research, housing, and job training for the brain-injured. In 1993, the most recent year for which statistics are available, the Bureau of Alcohol, Tobacco, and Firearms collected $7.7 billion in excise taxes on alcoholic beverages produced in the United States. Imagine what we could accomplish by doubling that tax alone. Spending just a quarter of the difference on helping victims of traumatic brain injury would generate a fund of $1.9 billion per year.

If the added expense occasioned by these taxes prompts people to drink less, drive fewer miles, or buy fewer guns, so much the better. Any reduction in high-risk activities means a drop in the number of associated traumatic brain injuries.

We have to do more than pay the cost. We have to retool our culture. We need to nurture rather than deny our impulses toward empathy, compassion, and fairness and restore these virtues as central values in our society.

The most effective, most rational way to halt the epidemic of traumatic brain injury is to dramatically reduce the number of brains that are damaged in the first place. That can be done. We could probably cut the incidence of severe brain trauma in half. Granted, we would have to agree to some tough trade-offs. And we would have to rethink our priorities. But if doing so would save thirty-five thousand to fifty thousand lives and prevent close to the same number of serious disabilities every year, wouldn't that be worth it?

Prevention: The Best Solution

No matter how much we improve our treatment of people with traumatic brain injuries and even if we took all the measures suggested in the previous chapter, obviously we would be better off if those 500,000 injuries a year never happened in the first place. Although we will never completely eliminate brain trauma, much of it is preventable, and the price of prevention is far less than the costs this epidemic imposes on us. For instance, in their 1989 report to Congress, *Cost of Injury in the United States,* Dorothy Rice, Ellen MacKenzie, and their colleagues estimated that after subtracting the price of the installation, putting dual air bags in every new car sold would save the country $4.7 billion in human capital over ten years. Fortunately, there are many practical steps like this that we can take.

Virtually every day, the media bring us stories of fatal accidents that should never have happened — accidents in which brain trauma is the cause of death, whether or not the reports mention that explicitly. An eighty-year-old woman loses control of her car, killing several pedestrians. A thirty-year-old man standing innocently on an inner-city street becomes the victim of a drive-by shooting aimed at someone in the building behind him. An inebriated twenty-three-year-old woman drives her pickup into a telephone pole, then dies from the resulting brain trauma. A motorcyclist skids on some gravel and falls, slamming his head on a curb; because he wasn't wearing a helmet, his injuries are fatal. A three-year-old girl dies because she wasn't strapped into a safety seat when the car in which she was a passenger collides with an eighteen-wheeler. A toddler in a wheeled walker is killed when he tumbles down a flight of stairs, landing on his head.

Tales of serious but nonfatal brain traumas, which occur far more frequently, often don't make the newspapers or broadcast news.

Consider the misery and money that we would save by cutting in half the number of Americans killed or severely disabled by brain trauma every year. About forty-five thousand people who would otherwise die would be alive and healthy; about forty thousand human beings who would otherwise be left with serious impairments would be whole. We would save $160 billion in lifetime costs for those who survive, not to mention the expense of futile trauma and acute care for those who don't.

We can do that. But it will take redesigning products that we use every day, making our built environment safer, enacting and enforcing laws and sanctions, voluntarily changing our behavior, and, most of all, altering our attitudes.

Lyndon Johnson once noted that each year more Americans were killed on the highway than died in the entire eleven years of the Vietnam War. Consider the turmoil and protest that single war caused with its forty-eight thousand American casualties. Many citizens, outraged by what seemed to be the senseless deaths of young soldiers, marched and petitioned until they forced a change in public policy and in cultural attitudes. A generation later, our nation's leaders still tread cautiously before involving the military in conflicts where American lives might be lost.

But every war has a purpose, however questionable or poorly articulated. The resulting deaths might not be worth the objective, but they aren't more meaningless than are most deaths from traumatic brain injury. Yet no one has marched on Washington to protest brain trauma. Brain injury isn't a hot topic among the politicians and pundits on the television talk shows that air every Sunday morning. We continue to quietly tolerate this tidal wave of destruction.

Perhaps one reason we fail to acknowledge it is that we don't really want to know. We don't want to concede that routine human activities, such as driving a car, are potentially so dangerous. We don't want to acknowledge that our casual attitudes toward alcohol, drugs, guns, aggression, and violence lie at the root of incidents that cause traumatic brain injury. In part, we don't want to know because we don't want to be afraid. In part, we already fear finding out what we don't want to know. Denial is motivated by fear, and fear reinforces denial.

We'll never eliminate traumatic brain injury entirely. That is a worthy ideal, but one we can only approach, never reach. Take Jeff Davis's accident, which I described in Chapter 6. Although Davis was wearing a helmet at the time, the spill he took while riding his bike down a gravel road sent him into a coma. The only way he could have avoided that injury would have been to refrain from rural cycling—an activity that gave him considerable pleasure and, when practiced safely, involves a relatively low level of risk.

While simply walking down a sidewalk, a person can be hit on the head by a flowerpot dislodged from a third-floor windowbox by the vibration of a passing truck. A driver operating a car at a normal rate of speed can hit a patch of black ice and spin into a light pole, which crashes through the driver's side window. About the only way we could assure complete safety from traumatic brain injury would be to buy a one-story house, pad the walls and counters, and stay inside. Even then, an earthquake might send our carefully constructed sanctuary tumbling down around our ears.

Few of us would be willing to go to such extremes to protect ourselves from head injury. That doesn't mean that we can't adopt less drastic methods for minimizing our individual risk and society's toll. For instance, for people sitting in the front seat during a car wreck, over-the-shoulder seat belts lower the risk of moderate to serious injury by 45 to 55 percent and the chance of death by 40 to 50 percent. Years of public information campaigns have bombarded us with these benefits, and using seat belts is mandatory in all but eight states. Nonetheless, in a survey reported by the National Highway and Traffic Safety Administration in 1995, only 68 percent of Americans buckle up. Sometimes it isn't that we don't know what will prevent injuries. We do know, but we just don't do it.

Published in 1989, the *Interagency Head Injury Task Force Report*, which was prepared by the Public Health Service, the National Institute of Health, and the National Institute of Neurological Disorders and Stroke, summed up a critical truth about brain trauma: "'Accidents' are often not chance or random events; instead, TBI [traumatic brain injury] generally occurs with great regularity to predictable portions of the population within specific settings. As a result, primary prevention efforts can focus on discrete changes needed to avoid brain injuries. Important advances have been made in the prevention of TBI in motor vehicle accidents through seat belt and helmet use, and installation of air bags. However, adoption of these and other equally effective methodologies is far less than optimal."

When it comes to taking personal action to prevent traumatic brain injury, what gets in our way is the value we place on individual freedom. In surveys reported in the journal *Science,* public health pundit Chauncey Starr found that Americans were willing to accept far higher levels of risk if they felt they had some degree of control over the situation. We all know people who feel comfortable driving long distances but are afraid of flying on a commercial airliner, even though statistically the plane is far safer. Often we're reluctant to let others impose on us a fraction of the danger that we freely take on ourselves.

Philosopher Geoffrey Rose expounds on a related obstacle, which he calls the "preventive paradox": "a preventive measure which brings much benefit to the population offers little to each participating individual." Each time I back out of my driveway, the chance of my being struck by another car is minuscule. Unless I indulge in unusually risky behavior, such as speeding or running red lights, that risk doesn't rise that much during the seven-mile drive to my office. But in my city of sixty thousand people, the likelihood of someone having a car wreck on any given day is fairly high, and a week seldom goes by without someone in town being killed or seriously brain-injured in an auto accident. If every one of us buckled up every time we got into a car, these wrecks might still occur, but the resulting injuries would be far less serious. In fact, public information campaigns need to stress this benefit more clearly. Some people still argue that they don't wear seat belts because they fear that the belts will cause internal injuries. If properly maintained and worn, belts are more likely to protect the chest and abdomen than harm them, but even a broken collarbone or bruised spleen is far less debilitating than a serious closed head injury.

It's often been noted that, as far as enlisting their patients in disease-prevention efforts goes, physicians have traditionally lagged far behind dentists, who for more than a generation have stressed the tooth-saving benefits of brushing, flossing, and fluoride. As the dangers of smoking, excessive alcohol, and cholesterol became widely publicized, many Americans gave up smoking, curtailed drinking, and changed their diets to include less meat and more fruits, vegetables, and grains. As the authors of *The New Medical Marketplace* observe, however, "the medical profession, . . . while formally advocating and applauding these changes, in actuality has done little to promote them." They continue, "Some feel that a major effort to ascertain, publicize, and diminish life-threatening habits may be the next significant step towards improving the human condition."

In fact, such an effort has already begun. The federal Centers for Disease Control and Prevention has designated ten injury prevention and research medical centers across the United States, including the one in Seattle that I discussed in Chapter 3. These centers study the causes and effects of specific injuries and then apply what they learn toward developing community programs that can stop injuries before they happen. Their association with medical centers bodes well for the future. Taught by professors who study and stress prevention, new physicians may become far more active than their predecessors were in helping patients, and thus society in general, stop brain trauma before it occurs by, for example, urging use of bike and equestrian helmets or mobilizing to lower highway speed limits.

Once health professionals are satisfied that they understand the who, what, where, when, why, and how of the various behaviors that lead to brain trauma and after they develop effective strategies to minimize them, the next step in prevention is launching full-scale public information campaigns. Everyone in the country should become fully aware of brain trauma, its causes, and what they can do to reduce the risk to themselves and their families.

Awareness alone can change behavior; sometimes a well-designed educational campaign is all it takes to prompt safer behavior. For instance, during the early 1980s, Los Angeles and Miami launched a blitz in schools and on television aimed at lowering the number of children darting out into traffic and being hit by cars. Using an animated character, the *Willy Whistle* program produced a 20 percent reduction in dart-out injuries and cut all child pedestrian injuries by 12 percent. A comparable campaign in Seattle elementary schools had similar positive results. Likewise, an Australian effort to encourage children to use bicycle helmets cut cycling injuries by 20 percent.

TAKING DRIVING SERIOUSLY

Next we must begin using sound public policy to attack the main culprits, beginning with motor vehicle accidents. Lowering the incidence of traumatic brain injury is a social challenge that demands reshaping our culture. We need to understand the potential benefits to us as individuals, but that isn't enough. A commitment to individualism has given America much that is unique and admirable, but in recent decades this commitment has evolved into a cult of individualism masking a growing tide of selfishness and self-indulgence. Nowhere is this more apparent than in our attitude toward motor vehicles. Virtually everywhere in the country except New York City, driving is such a routine daily activity for most people that we forget that it's the most dangerous thing most of us do. Since cars and motorcycles first hit the roadways in the late years of the last century, more than 3 million Americans have died in traffic accidents.

Every state should have laws requiring every adult occupant of a car, truck, or van—not just those in the front seat—to wear a properly functioning safety belt and every infant and child to be strapped into a car seat or other restraint appropriate to his or her age. And police in every state should be empowered to stop motorists for not using such restraints. Deaths of infants in traffic accidents dropped 37 percent between 1980 and 1984 as states enacted child restraint laws. No one should be allowed to ride in the back of a pickup truck unless he or she is strapped into a secured seat and the truck bed has a roll bar. Cars, trucks, and vans should be designed for safety. Every new one sold should have dual airbags, and manufacturers should make side panels, bumpers, and interiors that are better able to protect the people inside during collisions. We should adapt Canada's simple system for making vehicles easier to see: when a person turns on the ignition of any car, truck, or motorcycle sold in that country, the headlights go on. Norway and Sweden require daytime running lights on all vehicles. Since instituting that regulation in 1977, Sweden has seen an 11 percent drop in car accidents.

To encourage safer vehicles, the government could impose a surcharge on motorcycles and on cars and trucks that are less crashworthy and apply this money as rebates for the purchase of the cars that scored highest on safety.

Driving under the influence of alcohol or drugs should result in an immediate license suspension, whether or not an accident or injury occurs, and we should permanently take away the licenses of repeat offenders. The blood-alcohol level used to legally define intoxication should be dropped to the lowest level medically established as creating significant impairment, and it should be consistent in all states.

None of these regulations do much good if they aren't enforced, so we must give our law enforcement and regulatory agencies a clear mandate, insisting that they see to it that everyone complies. Fines should be set high enough to hurt, and license suspensions should be mandatory for dangerous violations.

Roads, bridges, and overpasses need to be redesigned so that they minimize the chance for accidents and lessen the potential for brain injury in the wrecks that do occur. For example, when public-works crews replace old lighting fixtures along thoroughfares, they should use the break-away light standards that can keep a one-car collision from becoming fatal.

Motorcyclists and their passengers must be required to wear helmets. The story of motorcycle helmet laws is one of the most bizarre episodes in our legislative history; it exemplifies the conflict between personal liberty and public good that underlies our collective paralysis in adopting policies that we know will prevent brain trauma. The epidemiological data clearly show that when helmet laws are in effect, motorcycle fatalities decrease. When the laws are repealed, as they were for a few years in California, fatalities and medical expenses rise. The costs of enforcing such laws are minuscule in proportion to the hospital bills, never mind the price of rehabilitation and lost potential, and since a higher than average percentage of motorcyclists are uninsured, the public shoulders most of the expense. Yet people continue to argue that requiring helmets impinges on inalienable rights.

In fact, we have no inalienable right to operate a vehicle on the public streets. Driving and cycling are privileges, and society can place on them any limitation that it deems to be in the public interest—provided that limitation is imposed equitably.

One limitation that we must place on driving is requiring that anyone who has been hospitalized for a traumatic brain injury pass both a rigorous cognitive assessment and a practical driving test before being allowed back behind the wheel or back on a motorcycle. Driving is a much more complex task than most of us recognize, and difficulty managing complex tasks is among the common deficits suffered by even the mildly brain-injured. One of the reasons for restricting the driving privileges of brain-trauma survivors is that even a minor reinjury can halt a promising recovery. But another is that a driver whose ability to process and respond to information is impaired is a threat to us all.

RAISING THE DRIVING AGE

Young drivers are another problem. Those under twenty-four account for close to half of all traffic fatalities, and teenagers, although representing only 7 percent of drivers, cause 13 percent of all collisions. For those between the ages of sixteen and eighteen, one-third of all deaths are from car crashes. In 1994 Senator John Danforth of Missouri and Congressman Frank Wolf of Virginia introduced the High-Risk Drivers Act, establishing a graduated licensing program; no one under eighteen could receive a full operator's license until he or she had maintained a violation-free driving record for one year. The bill also would promote more effective driver education and would set a blood-alcohol level of .02 — from one-quarter to one-fifth of the adult limit — as the level necessary to convict a person under twenty-one of driving under the influence.

The High-Risk Drivers Act failed to pass, and its chief sponsor, Senator Danforth, retired from the Senate at the end of 1994. But the bill did at least raise the issue of limiting driving privileges for those most at risk, and perhaps it will embolden some state legislatures to consider similar measures.

First implemented in New Zealand in 1987 and adopted in the Canadian provinces of Ontario and Nova Scotia in 1995, the concept of graduated licensing is to help sixteen-year-olds learn to drive in steps, lifting controls one by one as youngsters "graduate" to full licensing. Typically, the program limits at what times the teenagers may drive and with whom. It usually restricts new drivers to daylight hours; allows them to drive only with an older, experienced driver in the car; and limits the number of other teen passengers. In the United States only a few states have prohibited teenagers from driving during high-risk nighttime and early-morning hours.

Graduated driving provides the leverage that many parents would like to have in reining in teenage drivers. It recognizes that driving is a far more complex task than most sixteen-year-olds may appreciate. It gives the teenagers time not only to master skills but also to gain the maturity needed in operating a potentially lethal machine made of one and a half tons of metal and glass. And it ensures that by the time teenagers do hit the road at night with fellow teenagers, they will have gained sufficient on-road experience during the day.

While I accept the idea as a reasonable compromise, and while I recognize that it is the most that may be politically feasible right now, I don't think graduated licensing goes far enough. In my view, no one under eighteen should have a driver's license.

I grew up in the 1950s and 1960s, an era when teenagers could obtain drivers' licenses at an early age (I got mine at fifteen), drive cars without seat belts, and enjoy the mobility that automobiles provide. Back then I would have argued that freedom is worth the price. But now I'm older and wiser; having read the reports and studied the literature, I'm convinced that we have made a tragic social error by putting immature adolescents behind the wheels of deadly machines. During those first few years when I was driving, I was fortunate enough to avoid, but just barely, several wrecks which could have been serious, if not fatal. I don't think my experience was atypical.

An accident of American history put children behind the steering wheel almost as soon as they were tall enough to see over it and reach the gas and brake pedals at the same time. When cars and trucks became prevalent in the 1920s and 1930s, the country still had a large rural population. Older farm children had been driving the family wagon into town to sell produce or buy feed; it seemed to make sense for the kids to run the same chores in the new pickup or Model T. Driving also gave these adolescents welcome relief from the isolation of farm life and allowed them to socialize with their peers after school hours and in the summer. By the time their fathers and older brothers returned from World War II, American teenagers and their parents considered driving a basic right of high school students. It also made life much more convenient.

At least when the typical family owned only one automobile, fathers and mothers exercised some control over its use. But nowadays, working-class and middle-class households often own a motor vehicle for every adult. Among the affluent, a car has become a popular sixteenth birthday present.

Even if giving drivers' licenses to sixteen- and seventeen-year-olds had a sound basis two generations ago, it doesn't make sense anymore. Americans are overwhelmingly urban rather than rural. Yet we continue to license immature drivers out of habit and because we're not only eager to dispense with the responsibility of chauffeuring our kids but also reluctant to pay more taxes to make public transportation a viable alternative. This is neither necessary nor rational. Parents who didn't want to chauffeur their children to and from movies and football games and soccer practice could give them money for cabs. That would cost less than the hefty insurance penalty families pay for young drivers. Once we stop looking at driving as both a right and a rite of passage, once we view it clearly as a privilege entailing weighty responsibilities, we will begin to develop creative ways to make our teenagers as mobile as they reasonably need to be.

We protect our sons and daughters by not allowing them to serve in the military until they reach eighteen. Short of fighting in a war, driving a car may be the most dangerous thing they do in their entire lives. We can't afford to continue to treat it lightly. And we ought to be willing to tolerate the inconvenience and temporary conflicts that would result from making these rational changes, which would in fact protect all of us, including our young drivers.

High schools should stop conducting driver's education. Driver's ed classes may be intended to increase safety by teaching teenagers proper driving techniques, but ironically they decrease the overall level of safety by raising the number of young drivers on the road. No course can correct the immature judgment, recklessness, and vulnerability to peer pressure that afflicts adolescents. If the schools want to present a meaningful and appropriate course, they should teach bicycle and pedestrian safety, including the relevant traffic laws.

DRIVERS' EDUCATION FOR ADULTS

Taking driver's education out of the high schools doesn't mean that we would ignore it altogether. In fact, we should promote it—for adults. Insurance companies should be required to launch advertising campaigns stressing the savings that their customers would reap if they were to take defensive driving courses. Practical advanced driving courses should be developed and promoted, with even greater discounts on insurance premiums for those who take them. All beginning drivers should be required to take a rigorous driving course that emphasizes skills in responding to stress and dangerous situations; experience behind the wheel, not classroom time, is the key ingredient. In Britain, rigorous advanced driving tests have become quite trendy, with yuppies bragging over Brie about their scores. The London-based Institute of Advanced Motorists conducts a ninety-minute exam that includes maintaining a constant seventy miles per hour (the British speed limit) on motorways and passing slow traffic on winding country lanes. Drivers who pass get more than bragging rights; they can often receive a 30 percent discount on their insurance.

Above a certain age, a practical driving test shouldn't be optional; it should be an annual requirement for license renewal. Drivers over the age of sixty-five are involved in 10 percent of all accidents, and the main contributing factors are inattention, confusion, poor vision and hearing, and slow reflexes. The pace at which our faculties deteriorate as we get older varies from person to person. Some seventy-year-olds shouldn't be driving; some eighty-year-olds do fine. Periodic testing would flag these differences.

If the test were thorough enough, drivers who failed only one part of it could receive restricted licenses. For example, since night vision tends to deteriorate with age, a seventy-eight-year-old who could demonstrate safe driving before but not after dark should receive a license valid only during daylight hours. That way, that person could preserve the maximum amount of mobility and independence consistent with public safety.

Mandatory driving tests are fairer than other possible limitations on driving by the elderly, such as an automatic cutoff age, which wouldn't take individual variations into account. With America's baby boomers aging and life expectancy increasing, this country is faced with an ever-growing population of people who have depended on cars all their lives but whose abilities to drive safely are declining. We can't leave the decision about when to stop driving to individual judgment or depend on adult children to persuade their parents to hang up their car keys. To make the tests less burdensome and to identify younger drivers who might be similarly impaired, we could require practical driving tests every five years for drivers under fifty-five, every three years for those from fifty-five to seventy, and every year after that.

Motor vehicles are especially dangerous and destructive in the hands of reckless teenage males and octogenarians with impaired reflexes, vision, memory, and judgment. But they are potentially dangerous in anyone's hands, particularly when one is backing up or moving at fifty, sixty, or seventy miles per hour. Operating a car is increasingly perilous not only if one has taken certain medications or been drinking (and not just when one is drunk) but also when one is angry, distracted, or in a hurry.

We all recall times when we've had collisions or near misses because we failed to respect the fact that the automobiles we use every day may kill us and others. Compared to two-lane rural highways, freeways are relatively safe, but most of us have had close calls on interstate highways because another car was cutting in and out of traffic or was in our blind spot when we decided to change lanes. Crashes can and do occur—and quickly—simply because the driver's reflexes were a bit off or his or her attention wavered for a few seconds.

REDUCING OUR DEPENDENCE ON CARS

During the past two generations, cars have accustomed us to rushing from place to place far more than is necessary. We should all get into the habit of leaving for our destinations earlier and driving at no more than the speed limit. If we restrict the use of motor vehicles, we should provide reasonable alternatives. While people who won't be able to drive may not get around as quickly and conveniently as they do now, they will need transportation. Good bus and light rail systems, networks of hike and bike trails, and well-maintained sidewalks are essential.

All of this will cost money, but it will have the added benefit of reducing air pollution and promoting healthy exercise. New York manages to efficiently move millions of people around using the combinations of good sidewalks and good public transportation, even in a climate that is sometimes icy, sometimes wet, sometimes steamy. Copenhagen has one of the lowest rates of automobile ownership in Europe—just 228 cars per one thousand residents. In the city's commercial center, two-thirds of the people use buses and bicycles to get around. Instead of spending to build new roads, the Danish capital is funneling money to expanding and improving cycle and bus lanes.

AVOIDING FALLS

Public policy has less power when it comes to preventing falls, which cause 21 percent of all traumatic brain injuries. We can't reasonably pass laws prohibiting anyone under the age of four or over the age of sixty-five from living in a multistory house, but building codes do set standards for the design of stairs. These ordinances can be extended to require safety railings on apartment windows and on decks and outdoor landings. Public service campaigns can encourage parents of toddlers to use safety gates on stairs. Such modifications would prevent hundreds of children a year from falls like the one that I suffered when I was two.

The government could also offer tax breaks to landlords, the elderly, and parents of young children for safety modifications to dwellings. Sturdy hand rails on stairs, rounded edges on kitchen counters, nonskid surfaces on bathtub bottoms and shower floors can all save brains.

Among the elderly, alcohol is one of the biggest contributing factors to falls. As people age, their livers process alcohol less efficiently, so the ounce of eighty-proof whiskey that might not have affected one at forty can make one tipsy at seventy. Since balance, eyesight, and reflexes also decline with age, the chances increase that tipsiness may result in a stumble, and that the stumble may end in a fall. Many older people prudently cut down on their consumption of alcohol, but loneliness and depression lead some to drink even more than they did when they were younger. To combat the resulting number of falls and resultant brain injuries, we need a public service campaign urging the elderly to be moderate in their drinking—perhaps even to postpone their nightcaps until they're safely in their beds.

MAKING SPORTS SAFER

Sports and recreation accidents account for 10 percent of all brain trauma. Much of that could be eliminated if people wore appropriate helmets while participating in such risky activities as bicycling, skating, skateboarding, and horseback riding. Although bike helmets reduce the risk of brain injury by 88 percent, only an estimated 8 percent of riders wear them. When people engage in these activities on public streets and sidewalks or in public parks, we can enact—and enforce—ordinances requiring them to wear helmets. To encourage compliance under other circumstances, manufacturers can work on designing helmets with more comfort and visual appeal. Market-research focus groups could suggest the elements that would make helmets trendy: popular images, smart designs, or bright stripes in metal-flake paint could incline children and adolescents to put up less resistance to wearing helmets. Peer pressure exerts a powerful influence at those ages; no kid wants to look different. The more kids wear helmets, the more willing the rest will be to comply.

Certain sports gear actually causes head injuries. Surfboards propelled by powerful waves, for example, can deliver potentially lethal blows to swimmers, especially when the rider falls off and the board is out of control. To cut down on such damage, public beaches should segregate surfers from swimmers and require surfers to use the leashes many now use voluntarily in order to secure their boards to their ankles. Those ankle cords keep the board with the surfer when he or she falls off.

Some sports equipment is so inherently dangerous that it should be removed from the market altogether. Take lawn darts. Unlike the small darts used in the pub game, these are substantial projectiles tipped with pointed metal shafts several inches long. Thrown by someone with good upper-body strength, they hit the target with a force close to that of an arrow. When they miss, the results can be disastrous.

In April 1987, young Michelle Snow died in Riverside, California, after a lawn dart thrown by another child became embedded in her brain. Michelle's father, David Snow, lobbied the Consumer Product Safety Commission for a year and a half before convincing it to ban the sale of lawn darts. This was not, it turned out, an isolated case. The commission finally classified the dart not as a toy but as a dangerous object that has caused thousands of injuries, especially to children. But the Sporting Goods Manufacturers Association protested. In a statement reported in the October 29, 1988, *Houston Chronicle,* the trade group's director declared: "We felt that a ban is not warranted based on the limited number of fatalities associated with the product. . . . If used properly, the product poses no safety hazard, and . . . stronger enforcement by the commission could have corrected any distribution problem and not denied millions of Americans . . . years of recreational enjoyment."

Undoubtedly, the parents of Amy Herring were unpersuaded by the association's claims. The eleven-year-old Nashville girl was put into a deep coma after her cousin accidentally threw a lawn dart into her forehead. Doctors had induced the coma to prevent swelling after the eight hours of brain surgery required to remove the dart. Fortunately, lawn darts were taken off the market in 1988.

School, Pee-Wee League, and Little League coaches need to be especially aware of traumatic brain injury and what they can do to prevent it. Some level of indoctrination on brain and spinal cord injury, including meeting with survivors, should be a requirement for these positions. Not only would this make youth sports programs safer; it would also turn coaches, often children's favorite teachers, into influential advocates for brain-trauma prevention.

BANNING PRO BOXING

One sport—boxing—causes so much brain damage that it should be banned altogether. Short of that, it should at least be transformed completely. Brain injuries occur as a by-product of the intense physical confrontation inherent in American basketball, football, rugby, polo, and ice hockey. Even players of baseball, softball, soccer, tennis, racquetball, and squash may inadvertently suffer brain trauma. But only in boxing is the object of the contest to inflict traumatic brain injury on one's opponent. The most applauded achievement of a boxing match is a total knockout.

Numerous research studies have demonstrated that virtually all professional boxers suffer some degree of brain damage and that they are at much higher risk than the rest of the population for developing Alzheimer's disease. If repeated frequently, even mild brain trauma can add up to lasting disability. Boxing has recognized this by instituting protective headgear for boxers during practice, but that isn't enough, because the headgear comes off when the boxers enter the ring for real. Boxing gloves, while they reduce superficial cuts, actually increase the incidence of brain injuries because they allow fighters to hit harder without damaging their hands.

The only way to preserve the professional version of the sport while eliminating the devastation it causes is to change its object. Less vulnerable areas of the body could be identified and matches decided on the basis of who landed the most blows in those spots. Protective headgear should be required. That's what most countries have done for amateur matches; Sweden, that rational, safety-conscious country, has banned professional boxing altogether.

In football, the object is not to inflict injury on the opposing players; it is to carry the ball into the end zones. But the amount of mayhem that goes on in furthering that end has risen dramatically in recent years. Intentional helmet-to-helmet blows and other hits that can cause concussions have become commonplace in professional football since 1990, even though they're against the regulations of the National Football League. Even more alarming, 250,000 high school football players suffer concussions every year. Referees at all levels of the sport should come down hard on violations of any rule designed to prevent brain damage; players and even teams should be suspended after a stated number of infractions. Padded helmets designed to offer better protection are now on the market; anyone playing organized football should be required to wear one.

One disturbing trend in American athletics is the increase of violence in sports that don't necessarily entail it. Basketball, for instance, doesn't involve such outright sanctioned violence as tackling, yet kneeing, elbowing, and shoving have crept into the sport. Referees, who used to deliver swift and severe sanctions for such roughness, lately seem to be letting physical fouls slide. Maybe it's because fans find scuffles and falls exhilarating. As college and professional sports have become big entertainment business, players, coaches, and officials all seem to be pandering to this dark side of our natures. This has become so prevalent that during the 1994 playoffs of the National Basketball Association, television commentators wryly referred to the sport as "basket brawl."

College athletic conferences and professional leagues need to put a stop to this trend. Not only do violent athletes injure themselves and their fellows directly; because they serve as role models for so many youngsters as well as adults, they also help create and maintain a culture that considers violence permissible.

Certainly, our society must act quickly and decisively to control the assaults and other purposeful violence that result in 12 percent of all brain trauma. A majority of young children who suffer serious head injuries, 65 percent, are victims of child abuse—a tragic statistic. Some are punched with fists, hit with blunt objects, or thrown down stairs or against walls, but many receive their injuries when their parents shake them, in the mistaken assumption that shaking is a relatively harmless form of discipline. On the contrary, it can cause more damage than a blow, fall, or car accident, especially if repeated frequently. Every parent should be firmly informed of this hazard before taking a newborn home from the hospital.

We must strictly enforce existing laws to protect children from abuse. Any child whose abuse involves head trauma should be removed from the household immediately. Family counseling aimed at stopping abuse while keeping the family together is laudable, but traumatic brain injury is too serious for us to allow a child to remain in an environment where it might be repeated.

Finally, we must bite the bullet and outlaw the private possession of handguns and assault weapons. We've allowed the gun lobby to hold our common sense hostage for too long. As a defense against intruders, strong locks, loud dogs, well-placed motion-sensitive outdoor lighting, and functioning alarm systems work far better than does a pistol under a pillow or in a bedside drawer. Those who continue to feel insecure despite these precautions can carry cans of Mace, which can be a painfully effective defense weapon, especially at close range. Handguns are far more likely to kill their owners or members of their families than to stop a burglar or rapist. A handgun can provide protection only if it's accessible, and that almost always means having it within reach of children. Each year, scores of kids are killed playing with guns, and hundreds of suicides and domestic homicides are carried out with pistols their owners purchased to protect themselves and their families.

Arguments that we must arm ourselves to the teeth to protect ourselves from attack reflect our deep-seated ambivalence about violence. American culture not only tolerates violence; it reinforces and glorifies it. Our attitude toward violence is a mixture of fear, denial, attraction, and indifference. Violence is not merely endemic in American history; it is glorified in popular culture. We condemn violence, but at the same time we celebrate it. We love bellicose metaphors ("waging wars" on drugs and disease; "launching offensives" in politics). Movies and television dramatize our aggressive, destructive impulses and transform them into heroics. We fight violence with violence. By using the death penalty to murder murderers, we kill with premeditation those who kill others. We insist on the right to bear arms, even military assault weapons. Criminals use pistols and automatic rifles, children play with guns and knives, teenagers carry out contract killings, and the police and military display their weapons when they march in parades.

We extol those who use physical force to gain their ends, be they gangsters or sports heroes. We confuse power with domination. Television shows, movies, and news media relentlessly dramatize and report personal violence and war. But violent tendencies run deeper in the American consciousness and character. Freud believed that aggressiveness is a deeply rooted feature of human nature. Whether hostility, rage, and destructiveness are primary human characteristics or whether, as some modern psychologists believe, they result from deprivation and the frustration of basic needs, they play a leading role in human interaction. Freud was right when he declared that control of our aggressive impulses is absolutely essential to establishing and preserving civilization. Recurrent war is a constant threat to the fragile threads of civility that link nations. Recurrent interpersonal violence is a constant threat to civil order within nations and communities. And handguns are the most common instrument for wreaking irremediable interpersonal violence.

As troubling as violence itself is, our tolerance of violence may be an even more serious social problem. At the same time that we are arming ourselves, we continue in such high-risk behavior as driving after drinking or when we're tired. Violent death in car and motorcycle crashes, assaults, and falls, often involving alcohol or drugs, is an appallingly familiar feature of the American landscape. Yet gun fatalities may surpass traffic deaths by 2003. According to statistics released in 1994 by Secretary of Health and Human Services Donna Shalala, they already do in Texas and in five other states.

These two causes of devastating and often lethal brain trauma have much in common. Guns, knives, and clubs are instruments of violence; but so, potentially, are cars, trucks, and motorcycles. We don't ordinarily think of violence as a typical feature of the American highway, but it is. The pervasiveness of traffic violence may not show up directly in the injury and mortality statistics, but it is apparent in the behavior of drivers—in the reckless risk taking and outright hostility that we've all experienced on city streets as well as on freeways. You can see it in the drivers' eyes, their mouths, their gestures. You can hear it in the honking horns, the shouted curses. When some people get behind the wheel of a car, they become angry, aggressive, dangerous drivers. We have all had the experience of losing our tempers; when you lose your temper behind the wheel of a car, you become a threat to yourself and others. We have all felt frustrated by traffic or because we're late for an appointment; when you vent your frustration while driving a motor vehicle, you combine a dangerous instrument with a potentially lethal attitude. Given the increasing level of stress inherent in modern American life and our society's tolerance for aggression, it's a wonder that we don't see more car wrecks than we do. The occasional eruptions of freeway shootings by furious drivers are outrageous, but they are only the tip of an iceberg. Officials from the National Highway Traffic Safety Administration estimate that aggressive driving caused two-thirds of the forty-two thousand deaths on the highways in 1996. Three studies reported by the American Automobile Association cited "road rage" as a major cause of accident fatalities. The lack of common courtesy on the road is not simply aggravating; it is potentially deadly.

It's become fashionable lately to attack the frequent depiction of violence on television and in the movies, and there is some justification for the charges. Television and movies, after all, inevitably communicate values to the next generation. In September 1996, the American Medical Association announced that violent crime among children from thirteen to seventeen years old had climbed 126 percent from 1976 to 1992, and it argued, plausibly, that violence on television and in movies was partly to blame. The AMA also reported that it had commissioned a survey of eight hundred randomly selected voters nationwide and found a widespread public revulsion against media violence. "Fully two-thirds of all adults say they have turned off a television program or left a movie . . . that was too violent," the report accompanying the survey said; it added that 89 percent of women with children had done so. The pollsters further found that overwhelming majorities of parents wanted a stronger, more effective rating system for movies and similar rating system for television shows, computer games, and music. The data were used to buttress the AMA's then newly released *Physician Guide to Media Violence,* which it sent out to sixty thousand physicians, mostly pediatricians, and to every state attorney general. The guide included the following recommendations for parents: be alert to what shows their children are watching, keep televisions and vcrs out of children's bedrooms, avoid using the television set as a baby sitter, limit their own television viewing, and tell television sponsors and executives of their specific concerns about violence. The suggestions were at once obvious and, for many parents who had already ceded power over the channel changer to their children, far easier said than done. But although the media may pander to our attraction to violence, they don't entirely create it. Today's audience craves violence and will pay to witness it, just as the ancient Romans paid to watch gladiators fight each other or even wild animals to the death. Human beings are aggressive creatures who seek thrills, speed, and dominance. Violence toward others is one manifestation of these drives, and watching violent movies, television shows, or spectator sports allows us to experience this sense of excitement and power vicariously. Other cultures are able to refrain from using violence for entertainment, even though attraction to it seems to be a basic human quality. Examining the appeal that violence holds for Americans in particular may help us understand why we tolerate so much violent death and why we've done so little to reduce it.

Like our attitudes toward violence, our attitudes toward death are profoundly ambivalent. To avoid confronting death, we medicalize it. Driven by our crisis orientation and heroic impulses, we're comfortable dealing with death only when we're rescuing people from it. We've also become preoccupied with "death with dignity"—an ideal that few who leave this life achieve. We stress the domestication of death, as if everyone could remain lucid and free from pain to the end, without the mess of pressure sores and incontinence. Meanwhile, we avoid facing the fact that many thousands of people die violent, premature deaths that could have been avoided.

Prevention isn't always easy, but neither is it insurmountably difficult. Why, then, don't we do better?

One reason is that the American political process is slow. Numerous interest groups always adopt adversarial positions when confronted with proposed changes in the environment, in laws, and even in education. Thus, for example, driver's education teachers argue against eliminating driver's ed from the high school curriculum, even though data indicate that the courses do increase the numbers of sixteen- and seventeen-year-old drivers—a group that presents a high risk to themselves and to the rest of us. Why has it become an indicator of freedom in the United States that sixteen-year-olds are allowed to drive but not to vote? It would make much more sense to raise the driving age, setting both at eighteen. This approach to saving both lives and money seems so logical that it's almost unbelievable that there are no pressure groups introducing such measures. The evidence and arguments are available. What's lacking is the organized political voice to make them persuasive and have them heard and the political will to implement them.

Like typical adolescents, we cling tenaciously to the notion that violent death won't happen to us. This feeling isn't foolish. Some people *are* at greater risk of violent death—inexperienced, incompetent, intoxicated, frustrated, or harried drivers; angry gang members; armed robbers; police officers; soldiers in combat; anyone living or traveling in a region plagued by civil war or terrorism; combative males; depressed, indifferent females; children of abusive parents; individuals who drink heavily, use other mind-altering drugs, or suffer sensory or emotional disturbances. Still, most of the time, most people are at very little risk of death by violence.

But just as "it can't happen to me" may be true in general, "it can happen to anyone" may be true in a particular instance. Although the probability of a violent death may be low, the reality of it can erupt suddenly and unexpectedly. I still remember that when I was fourteen years old, one of my high school classmates was killed in a car crash on a curve that my friends and I had traversed thousands of times without mishap.

My classmate's death was a disaster. An untimely death always means a lost opportunity for a full, productive life. That loss has both economic and emotional dimensions. Family members lose a relationship that might have flourished, and they must deal with this irreversible loss for the rest of their own lives. Most of us can cope with loss, endure mourning, and go on. But the premature end of a life not yet lived troubles us especially and rekindles sadness every time we think about it. We must not inure ourselves to this genuine and appropriate response. We tend to turn away from these painful emotions, but we shouldn't, because in doing so we may also become even more tolerant of, perhaps even indifferent to, the violence that causes these deaths.

Some thinkers believe that human life has an intrinsic value—that it is valuable in itself. Many religions endorse a similar concept in advocating reverence for life, especially the life of a person or a potential person. I share the attraction to this idea of intrinsic value, sometimes to the point of yearning for a firm anchor—secular or religious—for its validity. Even if one remains doubtful that the intrinsic value of human life can be proven (in contrast to affirmed, accepted, or believed), it is a worthy idea. But the persistence of crime, aggression, ethnic hatred, and war undermines any illusion we might have that human beings share a consensus in favor of this notion. So does the prevalence of injuries that result, whether intentionally or unintentionally, from our aggressive impulses.

In America, we seem to value mobility, speed, and convenience more than we value human life. Mobility is an aspect of freedom; it frees us to travel, to explore, to discover new horizons. Speed allows us to do more sooner, thus further enhancing our freedom. Speed liberates, but it also kills. Combined with reckless abandon, speed propagates risk and often produces injury and death. Convenience, a particularly American obsession, is greatly enhanced by the automobile, truck, motorcycle, and bicycle. The convenient transportation of people and goods drives our "auto-erotic" culture. Every year, our addiction to mobility, speed, and convenience increases. Most of us can't imagine giving them up, or even compromising them for the sake of something we claim to value more.

If we sit down and examine the issue rationally, most of us would argue that we do place a higher value on human life than we do on mobility, speed, and convenience. It's just that we don't act as if we do.

One of the insane features of American culture is that we tolerate the violence caused by vehicular accidents, falls, blood sports, and assaults, while at the same time we advocate peace in the world. Peace on earth is an admirable goal but enormously difficult to achieve; prevention of brain injury in this country doesn't require international consensus. Think of what could be accomplished if the public, state and federal governments, and private organizations rallied around the common theme of brain-trauma prevention with the same kind of focused energy to injury prevention that we've brought to bear so successfully in the campaign against cigarettes. We wouldn't even have to wait for the long-term benefits, as we have in the antismoking effort; the benefits of preventing traumatic brain injury would be obvious and immediate.

We have the knowledge. Now we need to act. Most brain injuries can be prevented. The human and economic cost of injury can be reduced. All that's lacking is the collective will to do what has to be done.

Doing what we know we must to halt the epidemic of traumatic brain injury should begin with redirecting our culture away from violence and selfishness and toward civility and empathy. If we can accomplish that, the rational pragmatic steps will follow. We don't need to take every measure I've suggested in these last two chapters, but we do need to try some of them or develop alternative strategies. Other countries are far ahead of us; we can study what they have done and pick the best and most cost-effective approaches. Or we can look at measures that are working in some of our states and apply them nationwide. But we must begin to wake up from our long national slumber. We *can* curtail the brain-trauma epidemic. But we must first develop the national will to do it.

Bibliography

INTRODUCTION

For further information on traumatic brain injury, rehabilitation, and prevention, consult the following sites on the World Wide Web.

AAA Foundation	www.aaafts.org
Brain Injury Association	www.biausa.org
Neurotrauma–Law Nexus	www.neurolaw.com/brain.html
National Institute of Mental Health	www.nimh.nih.gov
WorldPath Internet Services	www.worldpath.net/~rboyce/brain.html

Fitzgerald, Dennis C. "Head Trauma: Hearing Loss and Dizziness." *Journal of Trauma: Injury, Infection, and Critical Care* 40 (1996): 488–496.

Shapiro, Kenneth. "Head Injury in Children." In *Central Nervous System Trauma Status Report,* ed. Donald P. Becker and John T. Povlishock. Bethesda, Md.: National Institute of Neurological and Communicative Disorders and Stroke, National Institutes of Health, 1985.

U.S. Department of Labor. Bureau of Labor Statistics. *Consumer Price Index*. Washington, D.C.: U.S. Government Printing Office, March 1997.

Wright, Barbara. *What Legislators Need to Know About Traumatic Brain Injury*. Denver and Washington, D.C.: National Conference of State Legislators, 1993.

CHAPTER 1: OUR VULNERABLE BRAINS

Andreasen, Nancy C. *The Broken Brain: The Biological Revolution in Psychiatry*. New York: Harper and Row, 1981.

Damasio, Antonio R. *Descartes' Error: Emotion, Reason, and the Human Brain*. New York: G. P. Putnam's Sons, 1994.

Damasio, Hanna, et al. "The Return of Phineas Gage: Clues About the Brain from the Skull of a Famous Patient." *Science* 264 (1994): 1102–1105.

Levin, Harvey S., Arthur L. Benton, and Robert G. Grossman. *Neurobehavioral Consequences of Closed Head Injury*. New York and Oxford: Oxford University Press, 1982.

Luria, A. R. *The Man with a Shattered World: The History of a Brain Wound*. Cambridge: Harvard University Press, 1972.

Restak, Richard M. *The Brain: The Last Frontier*. New York: Warner Books, 1979.

———. *The Modular Brain*. New York: Simon and Schuster, 1994.

Stein, Donald G., Simon Brailowsky, and Bruno Will. *Brain Repair*. New York and Oxford: Oxford University Press, 1995.

CHAPTER 2: SAVING LIVES

Colohan, Austin R. T., and N. M. Oyesiku. "Moderate Head Injury: An Overview." *Journal of Neurotrauma* 9, supp. 1 (1992): S259–S264.

Dickenson, Mollie. *Thumbs Up: The Life and Courageous Comeback of White House Press Secretary Jim Brady*. New York: William Morrow, 1987.

Eisenberg, Howard M. "Outcome After Head Injury: General Considerations and Neurobehavioral Recovery." In *Central Nervous System*

Trauma Status Report, ed. Donald P. Becker and John T. Povlishock. Bethesda, Md.: National Institute of Neurological and Communicative Disorders and Stroke, National Institutes of Health, 1985.

Hovda, David A., Donald P. Becker, and Yoichi Katayama. "Secondary Injury and Acidosis." *Journal of Neurotrauma* 9, supp. 1 (1992): S47–S60.

Miller, J. Douglas, Brian Pentland, and Sheldon Berrol. "Early Management and Evaluation." In *Rehabilitation of the Adult and Child with Traumatic Brain Injury,* ed. Mitchell Rosenthal et al. 2d ed. Philadelphia: F. A. Davis, 1990.

Nadeau, Robert L. *Mind, Machines, and Human Consciousness: Are There Limits to Artificial Intelligence?* Chicago: Contemporary Books, 1991.

Office of Scientific and Health Reports. National Institute of Neurological and Communicative Disorders and Stroke. *Head Injury: Hope Through Research.* Bethesda, Md.: National Institutes of Health, 1984.

Teasdale, G., E. Teasdale, and D. Hadley. "Computed Tomographic and Magnetic Resonance Imaging Classifications of Head Injury." *Journal of Neurotrauma* 9, supp. 1 (1992): S249–257.

Wright, Barbara. *What Legislators Need to Know About Traumatic Brain Injury.* Denver and Washington, D.C.: National Conference of State Legislators, 1993.

CHAPTER 3: HOPE ON THE HORIZON

Bedford, Patrick. "How the Airbag Shapes Your Information About Cars." *Car and Driver* 42 (June 1997): 20–21.

Eisenberg, Howard M., and Harvey S. Levin. "The Devastated Head Injury Patient." *Clinical Neurosurgery,* Congress of Neurological Surgeons 34 (1988): 572–586.

Gladwell, Malcolm. "Conquering the Coma." *New Yorker,* July 8, 1996, pp. 34–40.

Goldstein, Murray. "Traumatic Brain Injury: A Silent Epidemic." *Annals of Neurology* 27 (1990): 327.

Jacobs, Harvey E., Craig A. Muir, and James D. Cline. "Family Reactions to Persistent Vegetative State." *Journal of Head Trauma Rehabilitation* 1 (March 1986): 55–62.

Levin, H. S., et al. "Vegetative State After Closed-Head Injury: A Traumatic Coma Data Bank Report." *Archives of Neurology* 48 (1991): 580–585.

Office of Public Affairs. "UT-Houston Receives $7.2 Million to Study Hypothermia Treatment for Severe Traumatic Brain Injury." Press Release. The University of Texas-Houston Health Science Center, January 1995.

"Prayers for the 'Urgent Four.'" *New York Times,* July 4, 1996.

Traumatic Brain Injury Act, H.R. 248, 104th Cong., 2d Sess. (1995) (enacted as Public Law 104–166).

U.S. Department of Health and Human Services. "Injury-Control Recommendations: Bicycle Helmets." *Morbidity and Mortality Weekly Report* 44, no. RR-1 (1995): 1–13.

Wright, Barbara. *What Legislators Need to Know About Traumatic Brain Injury.* Denver and Washington, D.C.: National Conference of State Legislators, 1993.

CHAPTER 4: THE ROUGH ROAD TO REHABILITATION

Bates, Steve. "After Miracle, Brain-Injury Patient [Brian Rife] Struggles with Normal Life." *Washington Post,* September 5, 1994.

Blakely, James. "First Person Packet." Southborough, Mass.: National Head Injury Foundation, 1988.

Blow, Steve. "Therapist's Brain Injury Brings Insights." *Dallas Morning News,* June 30, 1993.

Boyer, Edward J. "Actor Gary Busey Critically Hurt in Culver City Motorcycle Crash." *Los Angeles Times,* December 5, 1988.

Braverman, Eric. "Healing the Brain." *Total Health* 14, no. 2 (1992): 55–56.

Burke, William H., Michael D. Wesolowski, and Mark L. Guth. "Comprehensive Head Injury Rehabilitation: An Outcome Evaluation." *Brain Injury* 2, no. 2 (1988): 313–322.

Caplan, Arthur L., Daniel Callahan, and Janet Haas. "Ethical and Policy

Issues in Rehabilitation Medicine." *Hastings Center Report* Special Supplement. Briarcliff Manor, N.Y., 1987.

Cole, James R., Nathan Cope, and Larry Cervelli. "Rehabilitation of the Severely Brain-Injured Patient: A Community-Based, Low-Cost Model Program." *Archives of Physical Medical Rehabilitation* 66 (1985): 38–40.

Cope, Nathan. "Neuropharmacologic Interventions in Traumatic Brain Injury." *Western Journal of Medicine* 153 (1990): 435.

Crisp, Ross. "Return to Work After Traumatic Brain Injury." *Journal of Rehabilitation* 58, no. 4 (1992): 27–33.

Dickenson, Mollie. *Thumbs Up: The Life and Courageous Comeback of White House Press Secretary Jim Brady.* New York: William Morrow, 1987.

Eagle, Kim. "Images in Clinical Medicine." *New England Journal of Medicine* 328 (1993): 620.

Geissen, Steve. "Isle Rehab Program Aiding Brain Injured Across the Nation." *Galveston Daily News,* August 20, 1989.

Golightly, Glen. "Miracle at Scarborough High: 'She Beat All of the Odds.'" *Houston Chronicle,* June 6, 1994.

Goshen-Gottstein, Esther. *Recalled to Life: The Story of a Coma.* New Haven: Yale University Press, 1988.

Haas, Janet F. "Admission to Rehabilitation Centers: Selection of Patients." *Archives of Physical Medical Rehabilitation* 69 (1988): 329–332.

Henry, Neil. "Patient No. 18,874: The Trauma of Brian Rife and His Family." *Washington Post,* June 11, 1986.

Hurt, Ginger D. "Mild Brain Injury: Critical Factors in Vocational Rehabilitation." *Journal of Rehabilitation* 57, no. 4 (1991): 36–40.

Karkabi, Barbara. "'Trying Like Hell': James S. Brady Retains Humor Despite Injury." *Houston Chronicle,* January 30, 1991.

Katz, Richard T., and John DeLuca. "Sequelae of Minor Traumatic Brain Injury." *American Family Physician* 46, no. 5 (1992): 1491–1498.

Kellerman, Frank R., and Tony Stankus. "Brain Injury and Rehabilitation." *Rehabilitation Quarterly* 28 (1988): 21–27.

Levine, Susan. "Head First." *Dallas Life Magazine* of the *Dallas Morning News,* February 16, 1992.

Linge, Frederick R. "What Does It Feel Like to Be Brain Damaged?" *Canada's Mental Health* 28, no. 3 (1980): 4–7.

Masters, Ardyce, and S. James Masters. "First Person Packet." Southborough, Mass.: National Head Injury Foundation, 1988.

McSherry, James A. "Cognitive Impairment After Head Injury." *American Family Physician* 40 (1989): 186–190.

Persinger, M. A. "Personality Changes Following Brain Injury as a Grief Response to the Loss of Sense of Self." *Psychological Reports* 72, no. 3 (1993): 1059–1068.

Rosen, Christine Duncan, and Joan P. Gerring. *Head Trauma: Educational Reintegration.* Boston: College-Hill Press, 1986.

Rosenthal, Mitchell, et al. *Rehabilitation of the Adult and Child with Traumatic Brain Injury.* 2d ed. Philadelphia: F. A. Davis, 1990.

Scofield, Giles R. "Ethical Considerations in Rehabilitation Medicine." *Archives of Physical Medicine and Rehabilitation* 74 (1993): 341–346.

Volpe, Bruce T., and Fletcher H. McDowell. "The Efficacy of Cognitive Rehabilitation in Patients with Traumatic Brain Injury." *Archives of Neurology* 47, no. 2 (1990): 220–222.

Wolcott, John. " 'Miracle' Mom and 'Miracle' Son Continue to Inspire." *National Right to Life News,* April 26, 1990, p. 15.

Wolpow, Edward R. "After the Fall: Mild Head Injury." *Harvard Health Letter* 16, no. 6 (1991): 1–3.

"Wounded Boy Recovering." *Houston Chronicle,* June 16, 1993.

CHAPTER 5: HOW FAMILIES BECOME VICTIMS

Brozan, Nadine. "Two Sides Are Bypassed in Lesbian Case." *New York Times,* April 26, 1991.

Burke, Emmie. "From One Family Member to Another." *Cognitive Rehabilitation* 2, no. 6 (1984): 16–19.

Burke, Michael. "Reflections of a Brother." *Cognitive Rehabilitation* 2, no. 3 (1984): 10–11.

Crisp, Ross. "Return to Work After Traumatic Brain Injury." *Journal of Rehabilitation* 58, no. 4 (1992): 27–34.

Jacobs, Harvey E., Craig A. Muir, and James D. Cline. "Family Reactions to Persistent Vegetative State." *Journal of Head Trauma Rehabilitation* 1 (1986): 55–62.

Kübler-Ross, Elisabeth. *On Death and Dying*. New York: Macmillan, 1969.

Levine, Susan. "Head First." *Dallas Life Magazine* of the *Dallas Morning News,* February 16, 1992.

Lezak, Muriel D. "Brain Damage Is a Family Affair." *Journal of Clinical and Experimental Neuropsychology* 10 (1988): 111–123.

Linge, Frederick R. "What Does It Feel Like to Be Brain Damaged?" *Canada's Mental Health* 28, no. 3 (1990): 4–7.

Masters, Ardyce, and S. James Masters. "Little Help." In "First Person Packet." Southborough, Mass.: National Head Injury Foundation, 1988.

Office of Scientific and Health Reports. National Institute of Neurological and Communicative Disorders and Stroke. *Head Injury: Hope Through Research*. Bethesda, Md.: National Institutes of Health, 1984.

Warrington, Janette Moffatt. *The Humpty Dumpty Syndrome*. Winona Lake, Ind.: Light and Life Press, 1981.

Wolpow, Edward R. "After the Fall: Mild Head Injury." *Harvard Health Letter* 16, no. 6 (1991): 1–3.

CHAPTER 6: FACING FATALITY—AND WORSE FATES

"Safest Teen Driver Apparently Asleep at Wheel in Crash." *Houston Post,* February 25, 1990.

Selzer, Richard. *Down from Troy: A Doctor Comes of Age*. New York: William Morrow, 1992.

Sosin, Daniel M., Jeffrey J. Sacks, and Suzanne M. Smith. "Head Injury: Associated Deaths in the United States from 1979 to 1986." *Journal of the American Medical Association* 262 (1989): 2251–2255.

Waxweiler, Richard J., et al. "Monitoring the Impact of Traumatic Brain Injury: A Review and Update." *Journal of Neurotrauma* 12 (1995): 509–526.

Kerr, Peter. "Centers for Head Injury Accused of Earning Millions for Neglect." *New York Times,* March 16, 1992.

Milz, Maggie. "Cost Containment and Accountability Factors." *Viewpoints* [Tangram Rehabilitation Network] 12 (1989): 2.

Morrison, Melissa. "Abuse Claims Close Home for Brain-Damaged Men." *Dallas Morning News,* July 11, 1993.

Mullins, Larry L. "Hate Revisited: Power, Envy, and Greed in the Rehabilitation Setting." *Archives of Physical Medicine and Rehabilitation* 70 (1989): 740–744.

Scofield, Giles R. "Ethical Considerations in Rehabilitation Medicine." *Archives of Physical Medicine and Rehabilitation* 74 (1993): 341–346.

Smith, Mark. "Texas Probe Zeros In on Rehab Centers." *Houston Chronicle,* March 29, 1992.

U.S. House. *Medicaid Brain Injury Rehabilitation Act of 1993.* 102d Cong., 1st sess., H.R. 2427. *Congressional Record* 139 (June 15, 1992): E1519–E1520.

U.S. House Committee on Government Operations; Human Resources and Intergovernmental Relations Subcommittee. *Rehabilitation Facilities for People with Head Injuries: Hearings Before the Human Resources and Intergovernmental Relations Subcommittee.* 102d Cong., 1st sess., February 19, 1992.

CHAPTER 8: A BETTER USE OF RESOURCES

Stoline, Anne M., and Jonathan P. Weiner. *The New Medical Marketplace: A Physician's Guide to the Health Care System in the 1990s.* 2d ed. Baltimore and London: Johns Hopkins University Press, 1993.

CHAPTER 9: POLICIES AND PRIORITIES

Alzheimer's Association. "1995 Statistical Fact Sheet."

Brody, Baruch A. "Justice in the Allocation of Public Resources to Disabled Citizens." *Archives of Physical Medicine and Rehabilitation* 69 (1988): 333–336.

Caplan, Arthur L., Daniel Callahan, and Janet Haas. "Ethical and Policy

Issues in Rehabilitation Medicine." *Hastings Center Report* Special Supplement. Briarcliff Manor, N.Y., 1987. Pp. 1–20.

Dyer, Keith E. "Head Injury: A Case Study and a Few of Its Medico-Legal Ramifications and Improvements Made." Paper written for medical jurisprudence course at University of Houston Law Center. October 8, 1988.

Frankowski, Ralph F. "Descriptive Epidemiologic Studies of Head Injury in the United States, 1974–1984." *Advances in Psychosomatic Medicine* 16 (1986): 153–172.

High, Walter M. Telephone interview, May 4, 1995, on outcome measures research at The Institute for Rehabilitation and Research (TIRR), where he is director of the Brain Injury Research Center.

Jones, Laurie. "Bill Aims to Curb Brain Injury." *American Medical News* 35, no. 39 (1992): 3–5.

Kennedy, Edward. Text of Senate Bill 725, presented to the U.S. Senate on April 1, 1993.

Kraus, Jess F., et al. "The Relationship of Family Income to the Incidence, External Causes, and Outcomes of Serious Brain Injury, San Diego County, California." *American Journal of Public Health* 76, no. 11 (1986): 1345–1347.

Lehmkuhl, Don. Telephone interview, May 5, 1995, on the work of TIRR's Research and Rehabilitation Training Center on Rehabilitation Interventions Following Traumatic Brain Injury, where he is director.

McMordie, William R., and Susan L. Barker. "The Financial Trauma of Head Injury." *Brain Injury* 2, no. 4 (1988): 357–364.

Muizelaar, J. Paul. "Adverse Effects of Prolonged Hyperventilation in Patients with Severe Head Injury." *Journal of the American Medical Association* 267 (1992): 1595.

National Advisory, Neurological Disorders and Stroke Council. *Progress and Promise: Status Report, Decade of the Brain.* Washington, D.C.: National Institute of Neurological Disorders and Stroke, National Institutes of Health, December 1992.

Noble, John H., et al. "Adequacy, Equity, and Efficiency in Managing the Behavioral Sequelae of Traumatic Brain Injury." Presented at the

National Conference on the Management of the Behavioral Sequelae of Traumatic Brain Injury, Arlington, Virginia, March 13–14, 1989.

Rice, Dorothy R., et al. "Cost of Injury in the United States: A Report to Congress, 1989." Produced for the National Highway Safety Administration, U.S. Department of Transportation, and the Centers for Disease Control, U.S. Department of Health and Human Services.

Shamberg, Shoshana. "Reentry Begins at Home: Maximizing Independence Through Environmental Modifications." *TBI Challenge!* winter 1994, pp. 4–8.

U.S. House. *Medicaid Brain Injury Rehabilitation Act of 1993.* 102d Cong., 1st sess., H.R. 2427. *Congressional Record* 139 (June 15, 1992): E1519–E1520.

Voelker, Rebecca. "Nineties Could See Brain Injury Reversal." *American Medical News,* December 22–29, 1989, p. 6.

Wright, Barbara. *What Legislators Need to Know About Traumatic Brain Injury.* Denver and Washington, D.C.: National Conference of State Legislators, 1993.

CHAPTER 10: PREVENTION

American Automobile Association Foundation for Traffic Safety. *Aggressive Driving: Three Studies.* Washington, D.C.: American Automobile Association Foundation, 1997.

American Medical Association. *Physician Guide to Media Violence.* Chicago: American Medical Association, 1996.

Associated Press. "Measure Would Forbid Children from Riding in Open Trucks." *Houston Chronicle,* December 19, 1994.

Baker, Sue. "Why Take an Advanced Driving Test?" *The Guardian,* July 23, 1994.

Beauchamp, Dan E. *The Health of the Republic: Epidemics, Medicine, and Moralism as Challenges to Democracy.* Philadelphia: Temple University Press, 1988.

Brody, Jane E. "Careless Divers Pay a High Price." *Houston Chronicle,* July 10, 1994.

Clark, A. J., and J. R. Sibert. "Why Child Cyclists Should Wear Helmets." *The Practitioner* 230 (1986): 513–514.

"Commission Bans Sale of 18-Inch Lawn Darts." *Houston Chronicle,* October 29, 1988.

Duhaime, Ann-Christine, et al. "The Shaken Baby Syndrome." *Journal of Neurosurgery* 66 (1987): 409–415.

Gusfield, Joseph R. *The Culture of Public Problems: Drinking, Driving, and the Symbolic Order.* Chicago: University of Chicago Press, 1981.

Institute of Medicine. *Disability in America: Toward a National Agenda for Prevention.* Washington, D.C.: National Academy Press, 1991.

Ivan, Leslie P. "The Impact of Head Trauma on Society." *Canadian Journal of Neurological Science* 11, no. 4 (1984): 417–420.

Jacobs, James B. *Drunk Driving: An American Dilemma.* Chicago and London, University of Chicago Press, 1989.

Jones, Ann. "Living with Guns, Playing with Fire." *Ms.* 4 (May 1994): 38–45.

King, Peter. "Halt the Head-Hunting." *Sports Illustrated,* December 19, 1994, pp. 26–37.

Knight, Robin, and Elizabeth De Bony. "Easing Gridlock, European Style." *U.S. News and World Report,* September 12, 1994, pp. 82–83.

Kriel, Robert L., et al. "Pediatric Head Injury Resulting from All-Terrain Vehicle Accidents." *Pediatrics* 78, no. 5 (1986): 933–935.

Leary, Warren E. "Head Injury Linked to Alzheimer's in Study." *New York Times,* March 1, 1990.

Lestina, Diane C., et al. "Motor Vehicle Crash Injury Patterns and the Virginia Seat Belt Law." *Journal of the American Medical Association* 265, no. 11 (1991): 1409–1413.

Linder, Stephen H. "Injury as Metaphor: Towards an Integration of Perspectives." *Accident Analysis and Prevention* 19, no. 1 (1987): 3–12.

O'Rourke, Nicolas A., et al. "Head Injuries to Children Riding Bicycles." *Medical Journal of Australia* 146 (1987): 619–621.

Public Health Service, National Institutes of Health, National Institute of Neurological Disorders and Stroke. *Interagency Head Injury Task Force*

Report. Washington, D.C.: Department of Health and Human Services, 1989.

Rice, Dorothy R., et al. "Cost of Injury in the United States: A Report to Congress, 1989." Produced for the National Highway Safety Administration, U.S. Department of Transportation, and the Centers for Disease Control, U.S. Department of Health and Human Services.

Robertson, Leon S. *Injury Epidemiology.* New York and Oxford: Oxford University Press, 1992.

Rose, Geoffrey. "Sick Individuals and Sick Populations." *International Journal of Epidemiology* 14 (1985): 32–38.

Starr, Chauncey. "Social Benefit Versus Technological Risk." *Science* 165 (1969): 1232–1238.

Stoline, Anne M., and Jonathan P. Weiner. *The New Medical Marketplace: A Physician's Guide to the Health Care System in the 1990s.* 2d ed. Baltimore and London: Johns Hopkins University Press, 1993.

U.S. Preventive Services Task Force. "Counseling to Prevent Motor Vehicle Injuries." *American Family Physician* 41 (1990): 1465–1470.

Van Buren, Abigail. "Safe Driver for Seventy Years Will Not Give Up Without a Fight," in "Dear Abby." *Galveston County Daily News,* December 23, 1994.

Weiss, Barry D. "Bicycle Helmet Use by Children." *Pediatrics* 77, no. 5 (1986).

Index

Rancho Los Amigos Cognitive Scale, 71–73

Reagan, Ronald, 7, 38, 68, 136

Rehabilitation: in United States, 11, 69, 125; and fraud, 125, 134, 137–138; centers, 127–128, 131–132, 139–140; and regulation, 134, 139–140, 165. *See also* Costs; Family; Therapy

Rife, Brian, 70–71

Rife, Janet, 71

Risker, Carlos, 73, 76

Rizek, David, 73–74

Robertson, Colman, and Stephens, 125–127, 128, 135

Rockefeller IV, Sen. John D., 139

Seat belts, 7, 52, 54, 178–179, 183

Sherman, Rosemarie, 123

Snow, David, 193

Snow, Michelle, 193

Spivack, Marilyn, 69

Sports injuries, 12, 156, 203; in boxing, 26, 174, 194; prevention of, 192–195; in basketball, 195

State governments, 173–174, 203

State laws: seat belts, 54, 178, 183; helmet, 56–57, 58, 60, 65; and Brain Injury Association, 69

Taxation, 173–174, 191

Texas Rehabilitation Commission, 174

Therapy: at Transitional Learning Community, 9, 76; rehabilitation and, 28, 133, 164, 173; hyperbaric, 48–49; speech, 77, 164; research in, 160, 162

Thompson, Karen, 102

Transitional Learning Community (TLC), 9, 76

Traumatic Brain Injury Act, 140

United States: fatality statistics in, 7, 11, 59, 106, 177; rehabilitation in, 11, 69, 125; costs of traumatic brain injury in, 11, 148–149, 155, 158; causes of traumatic brain injury in, 32–33, 54, 61; health care in, 43–44, 127–128, 171–174. *See also* Federal government

Vaiani, Al, 32, 33, 36

Vehicular accidents: statistics on, 10, 32; prevention of, 54–56, 178–179, 182–191; as cause of traumatic brain injury, 156, 174, 190, 198–199; costs of, 157. *See also* Driver's licenses; Seat belts

Violence, 21–33, 116, 156; prevention of, 13, 196–201; in media, 197, 199–200

Waldorf, Bobby, 150–152

Warrington, David, 100

Watts, Clark, 168–169

Winslade, William, 1–5

Zasler, Nathan, 131

Zazetsky, Leva, 15–17, 20, 25